DIABETES

Christopher D. Saudek, M.D.

and

Simeon Margolis, M.D., Ph.D.

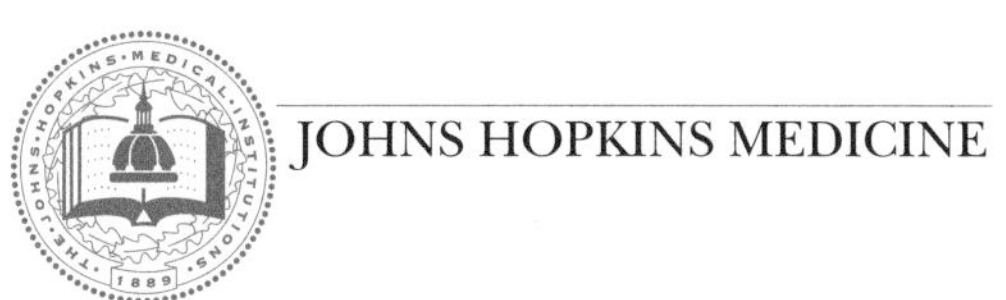

Dear Reader:

The number of people diagnosed with diabetes has increased dramatically in recent years. While there still is no cure for this serious condition, methods for monitoring and managing it have been significantly refined. People with diabetes now have the chance to live longer and healthier lives, and they can take advantage of advances such as less invasive blood glucose testing.

This White Paper reviews the most up-to-date information on the causes, symptoms, and advances in the treatment of both type 1 and type 2 diabetes—including insulin and oral drugs, lifestyle changes, and ways to reduce the risk of long-term complications.

Here are some of this year's highlights:

- Why some normal-weight people should worry about **body fat**. (page 12)
- The link between **TV watching** and diabetes. (page 13)
- What you need to know about **metabolic syndrome**, a common condition. (page 18)
- Should you be on a **low-glycemic-index diet**? (page 29)
- Surprising **benefits of pumping iron** for people with diabetes. (page 30)
- The latest research on **alcohol consumption** and blood glucose. (page 33)
- Should you try an **insulin pump** instead of insulin injections? (page 42)
- Intensive diabetes control benefits your **heart**. (page 53)

I hope that this knowledge will lead to more effective treatments and improve the quality of life of everyone with diabetes.

Sincerely,

Christopher D. Saudek, M.D.
Professor
Department of Medicine

P. S. Don't forget to visit www.HopkinsAfter50.com for the latest news on diabetes and other information that will complement your Johns Hopkins White Paper.

THE AUTHORS

Christopher D. Saudek, M.D., received his B.A. from Harvard University and his M.D. from Cornell University Medical College. He trained in internal medicine at Chicago's Presbyterian-St. Luke's Hospital and in metabolism at Boston City Hospital and Harvard Medical School. After serving on the faculty at Cornell and winning a Robert Wood Johnson Health Policy Fellowship, Dr. Saudek joined the faculty of the Johns Hopkins University School of Medicine, where he is currently professor of medicine, director of the Johns Hopkins Diabetes Center, and director of the General Clinical Research Center.

A past president of the American Diabetes Association, Dr. Saudek is active in diabetes education and public health policy. His research focuses on the development of an implantable insulin pump, a topic on which he has published widely. He is author of *The Johns Hopkins Guide to Diabetes: For Today and Tomorrow.* In 1991, he was named Outstanding Clinician in Diabetes by the American Diabetes Association.

▪ ▪ ▪

Simeon Margolis, M.D., Ph.D., received his M.D. and Ph.D. from the Johns Hopkins University School of Medicine and performed his internship and residency at Johns Hopkins Hospital. He is currently a professor of medicine and biological chemistry at the Johns Hopkins University School of Medicine and medical editor of *The Johns Hopkins Medical Letter: Health After 50.* He has served on various committees for the Department of Health, Education, and Welfare, including the National Diabetes Advisory Board and the Arteriosclerosis Specialized Centers of Research Review Committees. In addition, he has acted as a member of the Endocrinology and Metabolism Panel of the U.S. Food and Drug Administration.

A former weekly columnist for *The Baltimore Sun,* Dr. Margolis lectures regularly to medical students, physicians, and the general public on a wide variety of topics, such as the prevention of coronary heart disease, the control of cholesterol levels, the treatment of diabetes, and the use of alternative medicine.

CONTENTS

DIABETES

Diabetes mellitus, also referred to simply as diabetes, is a metabolic disorder characterized by abnormally high levels of glucose (sugar) in the blood. The disorder occurs when the body's production of insulin is inadequate or its response to insulin is insufficient. Insulin is a hormone that controls the production of glucose by the liver and allows cells to remove glucose from the blood.

The term "diabetes mellitus" is derived from the Greek word for siphon and the Latin word *mellitus,* meaning honey-sweet. The disease is aptly named because the excretion of large amounts of sugar-laden urine is a key manifestation of poorly controlled diabetes. The two principal dangers for people with diabetes are the immediate complications of high blood glucose levels and the long-term complications affecting the eyes, nerves, kidneys, and large blood vessels.

PREVALENCE OF DIABETES

In the United States, the prevalence of diabetes currently stands at about 17 million people, about a third of whom do not yet know they have the disease. A large portion, some 7 million, are age 65 or older. Since 1990, the number of people diagnosed with diabetes has increased considerably, rising from less than 5% of Americans to about 8% today. In 2000, an estimated 1 million new cases of diabetes were diagnosed.

TYPES OF DIABETES

Diabetes is divided into two types. Type 1 diabetes usually arises before age 30 and tends to come on suddenly. Type 2 diabetes, which accounts for 90% to 95% of diabetes cases, usually starts later in life. The onset of type 2 diabetes tends to be more gradual, and blood glucose levels are more stable. Most people with type 2 diabetes are obese.

Type 1 diabetes was once called insulin-dependent or juvenile diabetes; type 2 diabetes was known as non-insulin-dependent or adult-onset diabetes. These terms are no longer used because some people with type 2 diabetes eventually require treatment with insulin and there is a growing epidemic of type 2 disease in children.

PRE-DIABETES

Pre-diabetes is a new term used to describe a medical condition whereby blood glucose levels are higher than normal but not high enough to be diagnostic of diabetes. Names previously used for the condition were impaired fasting glucose and impaired glucose tolerance. About 12 million Americans between the ages of 45 and 74 have pre-diabetes. Without treatment, most of them will develop type 2 diabetes within 10 years.

CAUSES OF DIABETES

Diabetes is caused by an abnormality in the way the body uses glucose. This abnormality results from insufficient production of insulin by the pancreas, resistance of the body's tissues to insulin action, or a combination of both.

Each cell in the body needs a regular supply of glucose, which enters the bloodstream from the digestion and absorption of dietary carbohydrates or from the liver where it is produced. When enough insulin is present in the blood, the liver shuts down its production of glucose and glucose in the blood enters cells. Some of the glucose is used immediately by the cells as a source of energy; most of the rest is converted to glycogen in the liver and muscles, where it is stored for future use. The body's ability to store glycogen is limited, however. Glucose not used immediately for energy or stored as glycogen is converted to triglycerides and stored in adipose (fat) tissue.

Insulin—a hormone produced by beta cells in a part of the pancreas known as the islets of Langerhans—is the key regulator of glucose uptake by muscle and fat. As blood glucose levels rise after a meal, the pancreas responds by secreting insulin into the bloodstream. Insulin attaches to receptor sites on the surface of cells throughout the body. By a complex series of events, the binding of insulin to these receptors causes carrier proteins, called glucose transport proteins, to move from inside the cell to the cell's surface. Like little dump trucks, these glucose transport proteins deliver glucose from outside the cell to the inside. But without the initial binding of insulin to receptors on the cell's surface, glucose cannot enter cells.

Insulin also plays a role in preventing excessive release of glucose from the liver into the bloodstream between meals. Pancreatic cells in the islets of Langerhans continuously monitor blood glucose levels and release insulin or glucagon as needed. (Glucagon is

How the Pancreas Regulates Blood Glucose

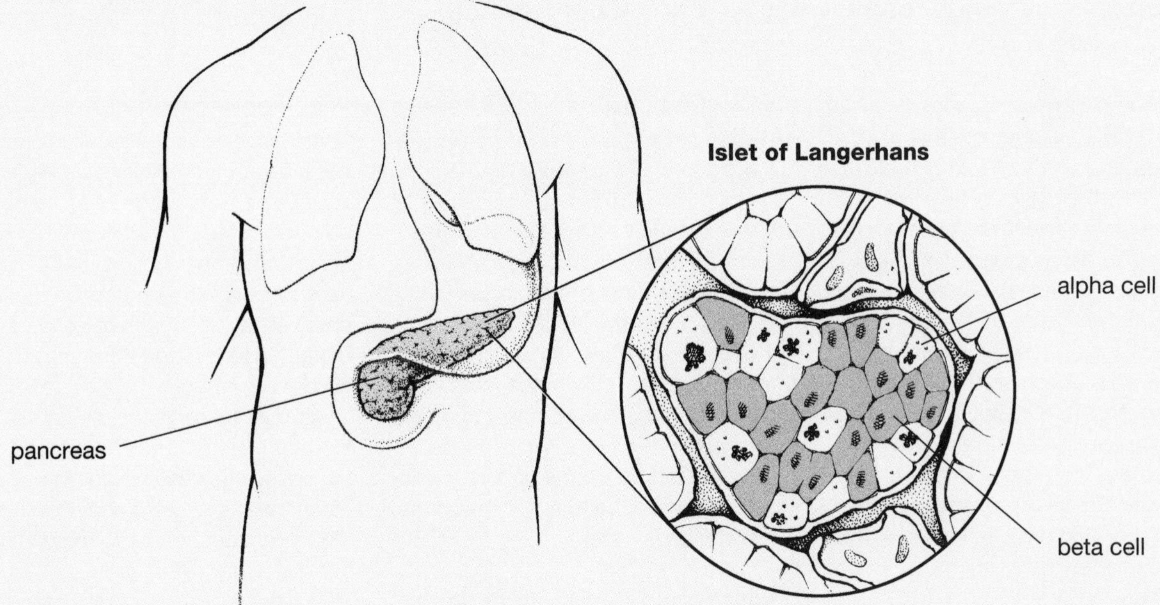

The pancreas is an elongated organ that extends across the abdomen, below the stomach. In addition to secreting certain enzymes that aid in food digestion, the pancreas also manufactures hormones responsible for regulating blood glucose levels. Scattered throughout the pancreas are more than a million tiny nests of cells known as the islets of Langerhans. Each islet contains several different types of cells. The majority are beta cells, which produce and store the hormone insulin until it is needed. Also located in the islets are alpha cells, which make and store glucagon, a hormone that counteracts the effects of insulin.

After a meal, the carbohydrates in foods are converted into glucose and enter the bloodstream. Beta cells sense the rising blood glucose levels and secrete insulin into the blood. Once in the bloodstream, insulin helps glucose enter the body's cells, where it is "burned" for energy or converted to glycogen by the liver and muscles and stored there for future energy needs. As a result, blood glucose levels return to normal, and insulin secretion decreases.

On the other hand, a drop in blood glucose levels—for example, when one hasn't eaten for several hours—stimulates the alpha cells to secrete glucagon into the blood. Glucagon raises blood glucose levels by signaling the liver to convert stored glycogen back into glucose and release it into the bloodstream.

Normally, the secretion of these hormones by the pancreas is perfectly balanced: Beta and alpha cells continuously monitor blood glucose levels and release insulin or glucagon as needed. In diabetes, this balance is impaired because the beta cells produce little or no insulin, the body's cells are resistant to insulin, or a combination of both is at work. Regardless, glucose cannot enter cells effectively and remains in the bloodstream. The result is persistently high blood glucose levels (hyperglycemia). Without treatment, hyperglycemia can lead to serious long-term complications, such as heart, eye, and kidney disease.

a hormone that raises blood glucose levels by signaling the liver to convert amino acids and glycogen to glucose and to send the glucose into the bloodstream.) In diabetes, the balance between insulin and glucagon is disrupted either by insufficient insulin production or insulin resistance; the result is elevated blood glucose levels.

Causes of type 1 diabetes. Type 1 diabetes is an autoimmune disease: The body produces antibodies that attack and damage beta

Why Does Obesity Contribute to Diabetes?

Excess body weight can lower your body's sensitivity to insulin and make you more susceptible to type 2 diabetes.

Obesity is the most important risk factor for type 2 diabetes. Extremely obese people (those with a body mass index [BMI] of 40 or greater) are seven times more likely than normal-weight people to develop type 2 diabetes.

As obesity has become more common in the United States, so has type 2 diabetes. In 1991, 12% of Americans were obese and 5% had diabetes. By 2001, nearly 21% of Americans were obese and 8% had diabetes. The reason why obesity increases the risk of diabetes is not clearly understood, but several possible explanations exist.

Obesity and Insulin

Type 2 diabetes involves a two-step process that first affects the body's response to, and later its production of, insulin. The decreased responsiveness to insulin, called insulin resistance, forces the pancreas to work harder and produce more insulin. The pancreas of a normal-weight person might put out 30 units of insulin a day. If that person becomes obese, those same 30 units are no longer sufficient to clear glucose from the bloodstream, and more insulin is required. The pancreas starts to produce more insulin to keep up with the increased demand, but not everyone's pancreas can handle the extra workload. Diabetes results when the pancreas cannot produce enough insulin to control blood glucose levels.

Why Some Overweight People Don't Have Diabetes

Having a high BMI, a measure of body fat based on both height and weight, increases the risk of having diabetes. People with a BMI of 25 to 29.9 are considered overweight, and those with a BMI of 30 or above are considered obese. Although most people with type 2 diabetes (80%) are obese, most obese people don't have diabetes—so other factors clearly are at work. Most likely, genes determine whether someone's pancreas is hardy enough to produce the extra insulin needed if the person becomes overweight.

Another factor is the distribution of the extra weight. People with abdominal obesity (excess weight above the hips) are more likely to develop type 2 diabetes than those with extra weight in the hips and thighs.

Abdominal obesity and elevated blood glucose levels are two components of metabolic syndrome, a cluster of findings present in about one out of four Americans that increases the risk of diabetes, as well as the risk of coronary heart disease and stroke.

cells in the pancreas that secrete insulin. At first, the ability of the beta cells to produce insulin is merely impaired, but eventually (usually in less than a year) the cells produce little or no insulin. Fortunately, the body's cells still respond normally to insulin, so people with type 1 diabetes can compensate for the lack of insulin with insulin injections. Although heredity plays some role in type 1 diabetes, most patients have no family history of diabetes.

Causes of type 2 diabetes. Type 2 diabetes is caused by a combination of insulin resistance (reduced sensitivity of the body's tissues, primarily the liver and muscles, to the action of insulin) and inadequate amounts of insulin. In people with insulin resistance, the pancreas must increase its production of insulin so that cells can get the glucose they need. Diabetes results when the pancreas is unable to secrete enough extra insulin to overcome the tissue resistance. The majority of people with type 2 diabetes can be treated with lifestyle measures (diet and exercise) or oral medications, but about 40% need insulin injections to achieve adequate control of their blood glucose.

(For more on metabolic syndrome, see the feature on pages 18–19.)

New Findings on Obesity and Diabetes

New theories have emerged recently about the possible links between obesity and diabetes. For example, experts have found that fat cells secrete many hormone-like substances that circulate through the bloodstream and can affect other systems in the body. Recent research has focused on three substances produced by fat cells: resistin, leptin, and free fatty acids.

Resistin. In 2001, researchers published a study in *Nature* describing a previously unknown hormone called resistin that, in mice, appeared to increase with greater body weight. The researchers found that higher blood levels of resistin led to insulin resistance, and antibodies that blocked resistin improved insulin sensitivity. They discovered that several diabetes drugs already in use work in part by blocking the gene that makes resistin. Now, researchers are investigating whether a drug that specifically targets resistin can help improve insulin sensitivity with fewer side effects.

Leptin. Leptin, first discovered in 1994, is a hormone that signals the brain that no more food is needed—it has been referred to as an appetite suppressant or "satiety signal." Obese people have high blood levels of leptin, so researchers speculate that they may not be sensitive to the appetite and weight suppression that leptin ordinarily provides. The role that leptin plays in appetite is not yet fully understood, but further research may lead to new targets for obesity and diabetes drugs.

Free fatty acids. Free fatty acids, which are formed from the breakdown of stored fat in fat cells, circulate through the body and may also contribute to insulin resistance and type 2 diabetes. Normally, muscle cells remove glucose from the bloodstream for use as energy. However, research suggests that accumulation of fatty acids in muscle cells of obese people may prevent glucose from entering these cells. The resulting rise in blood glucose levels is the main characteristic of diabetes.

Positive Results

The good news is that type 2 diabetes is very sensitive to weight loss and occasionally may disappear when obese people lose weight. Weight loss should be achieved through a combination of increased physical activity and reduced calorie intake. Improved insulin resistance can occur with a loss of as few as 5 lbs., but better results are achieved with a 7% to 15% decrease in body weight. In 2002, the Diabetes Prevention Program study showed that people who followed a low-calorie, low-fat diet; exercised 30 minutes a day; and lost an average of 15 lbs. were 58% less likely to develop type 2 diabetes over a three-year period than people who took a placebo pill.

Obesity is a major contributing factor to insulin resistance and type 2 diabetes. About 80% of people with type 2 diabetes are obese, and the risk of type 2 diabetes rises as a person's weight increases. To learn why obesity increases the risk of diabetes, see the feature above.

Heredity also plays an important role in type 2 diabetes. In a study of more than 200 people with type 2 diabetes (age 35 to 74), 66% reported at least one relative with diabetes and 46% had at least two relatives with the disease. In particular, people whose mother had diabetes were two times more likely to get the disease than those whose father had it—33% vs. 17%. Of the women with diabetes, 11% had at least one child with diabetes, whereas only 4% of the men with diabetes had a child with the disorder.

Other causes of diabetes. A small number of people develop diabetes because they have another disorder. For example, diabetes can result from diseases that destroy the pancreas—such as hemochromatosis (excessive absorption and storage of iron) or chronic pancreatitis (inflammation of the pancreas)—or from surgical removal of the pancreas, for instance, in people with pancreatic cancer. Tumors of certain organs can cause diabetes as a result of overproduction of hormones that interfere with insulin action. For example, growth hormone produced by some tumors of the pituitary gland, cortisol or epinephrine from adrenal tumors, and glucagon from pancreatic tumors can all raise blood glucose levels. Corticosteroids, commonly used to treat asthma and arthritis, and thiazide diuretics, typically used in the treatment of high blood pressure and heart failure, may also bring on diabetes in people who are predisposed to the illness.

PREVENTION OF DIABETES

Although researchers have been unable to identify ways to prevent type 1 diabetes, people can take measures to reduce their risk of type 2 disease.

Prevention of type 1 diabetes. The Diabetes Prevention Trial—Type 1 looked at whether insulin injections or oral insulin might prevent type 1 diabetes in people at increased risk for the disease. The results revealed that neither treatment protects against the disease. Other researchers have studied immunosuppressive drugs for the prevention of type 1 diabetes, but the results have not been encouraging.

Prevention of type 2 diabetes. Efforts to prevent type 2 diabetes are especially important for people at high risk for developing the disease—those who have pre-diabetes, are overweight, have a family history of the disorder, belong to a high-risk ethnic group (such as blacks, Hispanics, Asians, or Native Americans), or have a history of diabetes during pregnancy (gestational diabetes).

The Diabetes Prevention Program study found that people with pre-diabetes can take steps to prevent type 2 diabetes. In the study, participants who followed a low-calorie, low-fat diet; exercised 30 minutes a day; and lost an average of 15 lbs. were 58% less likely to develop type 2 diabetes over a three-year period than people who did not make these lifestyle changes. In addition, people who took the diabetes drug metformin (Glucophage) reduced their risk of type 2 diabetes by 31%, compared with people who received a placebo. In another study, the Heart Outcomes Prevention Evaluation (HOPE), people taking the ACE inhibitor ramipril (Altace) were 30% less likely to develop diabetes than those taking a placebo.

In addition, a high-fiber diet may decrease the risk of developing type 2 diabetes. An observational study of nearly 36,000 women

NEW RESEARCH

Americans Have a 1 in 3 Chance of Developing Diabetes

Lifetime risks have been established for a number of disorders, but the lifetime risk of diabetes in the United States was not known. Now, a study finds that people born in the United States in 2000 have a 1 in 3 chance of being diagnosed with diabetes at some point in their lives.

Researchers used data from a 16-year health survey of more than 350,000 people. They found that the risk of diabetes is higher among women than men at every age, and that the estimated lifetime risk is higher among minorities than among whites. (For example, the estimated lifetime risk for Hispanic men and women is about 50%.)

Diabetes also has a significant impact on early death and quality of life. For example, a man diagnosed with diabetes at age 40 will live 12 years less than a similar man without diabetes, and will have a 19-year decrease in quality-of-life years.

The researchers point out that Americans are more likely to have diabetes than most other health conditions. "For example, the lifetime risk of diabetes is considerably higher than the widely publicized 1 in 8 risk for breast cancer among U.S. women," they write.

JOURNAL OF THE AMERICAN MEDICAL ASSOCIATION
Volume 290, page 1884
October 8, 2003

found that those who consumed the most fiber from cereal had a 36% lower risk of developing type 2 diabetes than those consuming the least fiber from cereal. A more recent study from Finland reported similar results in men and women (see the sidebar on page 27).

Finally, quitting smoking may reduce the risk of type 2 diabetes. A study of more than 21,000 U.S. male physicians found that those who smoked 20 or more cigarettes a day were 70% more likely to develop diabetes than those who had never smoked or were former smokers.

ACUTE SYMPTOMS OF DIABETES

The initial symptoms of diabetes are usually related to hyperglycemia, the medical term for high blood glucose. The onset of type 1 diabetes is often sudden, and diabetic ketoacidosis (see page 8) may be the first indication of the disease. In contrast, type 2 diabetes usually develops gradually, and some people experience few or no symptoms for a number of years. In these individuals, chronic diabetes complications, such as peripheral neuropathy (nerve damage in the hands or feet) or coronary heart disease (CHD), may be the first indication of diabetes. In other people without symptoms, the diagnosis of type 2 diabetes is made after a routine laboratory test.

Classic presenting symptoms. The classic presenting symptoms of diabetes are an increased frequency of urination (polyuria), increased thirst and fluid intake (polydipsia), and, as the disease progresses, weight loss despite increased hunger and food intake (polyphagia). These symptoms are caused by high blood glucose and the resulting "spillover" of excess glucose into the urine; they can be prevented by maintaining reasonable blood glucose levels.

Other common symptoms of diabetes include blurred vision due to changing levels of glucose in the eye; weakness and fatigue; recurrent vaginal yeast infections; and skin infections. These symptoms are transient, do not indicate any permanent damage, and can be eliminated by controlling blood glucose levels.

When people receiving treatment for diabetes experience symptoms of high blood glucose, they need to contact their doctor to determine whether their treatment regimen needs to be adjusted. For example, people with type 2 diabetes who are using exercise and diet alone to control blood glucose levels may need to start taking oral medications or insulin. People already taking oral medications or insulin may need to increase the dosage. In either case, people

NEW RESEARCH

Obesity, Diabetes Rates Rise Again

Continuing a trend that began in the 1990s, the percentage of people in the United States who are obese or have diabetes rose in 2001, investigators from the Centers for Disease Control and Prevention report.

In 2001, nearly 21% of adults (44.3 million Americans) were obese (i.e., a body mass index [BMI] of 30 or greater), up from 20% in 2000 and 12% in 1991. Also, about 2% of the U.S. adult population was morbidly obese (a BMI of 40 or greater) in 2001. Obesity significantly increases the risk of diabetes, high blood pressure, arthritis, asthma, and high cholesterol. Diabetes was diagnosed in about 8% of American adults in 2001, up from 7% in 2000 and 5% in 1991.

Researchers conducted telephone interviews with 195,005 Americans age 18 and older. Because people often underestimate their weight and overestimate their height, the actual rates of obesity are likely much higher. A recent study that measured people's weight and height, rather than using self-reports, found an obesity rate of 30%. The diabetes rate may also be too low, since about 35% of diabetes cases are undiagnosed.

Programs to "promote a balanced diet, increase physical activity, and maintain weight control must be national priorities," the researchers write.

JOURNAL OF THE AMERICAN MEDICAL ASSOCIATION
Volume 289, page 76
January 1, 2003

with diabetes should follow their prescribed treatment plan carefully to achieve optimal blood glucose control.

Diabetic ketoacidosis. This acute complication of diabetes results when a nearly complete lack of insulin forces the body to utilize sources of energy other than glucose—namely, fatty acids released from fat tissue. These fatty acids are broken down by the liver into compounds known as ketone bodies. The accumulation of ketone bodies increases the acidity of the blood to dangerous levels, a condition called metabolic acidosis.

In addition, elevated blood glucose levels (above 200 mg/dL) due to the lack of insulin leads to the excretion of large amounts of glucose and water in the urine, causing severe dehydration. Diabetic ketoacidosis typically occurs only in people who have type 1 diabetes, but it can occasionally occur in those with type 2 diabetes if they are under physical stress—for example, after a stroke or when fighting an infection.

For a list of the symptoms of ketoacidosis and what to do if they occur, see the feature on the opposite page.

Hyperosmolar nonketotic state. The stress of an injury or major illness, such as a stroke, heart attack, or severe infection, can raise blood glucose to extremely high levels in people with type 2 diabetes. While insulin levels are adequate to avert excessive ketone body production, they are not high enough to prevent high blood glucose levels and the rise in blood osmolarity (thickness) that gives the condition its name. In about a third of people who experience hyperosmolar state, the condition is the first indication that they have diabetes.

For a list of the symptoms of hyperosmolar state and what to do if they occur, see the feature on the opposite page.

DIAGNOSIS AND OFFICE FOLLOW-UP OF DIABETES

Certain symptoms suggest the presence of diabetes, but laboratory tests are needed to make the diagnosis. In an effort to promote the early detection of diabetes and reduce the risk of long-term complications, the American Diabetes Association recommends that people age 45 and older be tested for the disease every three years.

People at elevated risk for diabetes, however, should be tested before age 45 and more frequently (for example, every one to two years). These people include those who are obese; have a first-degree relative (parent or sibling) with diabetes; belong to a high-risk ethnic group (including blacks, Hispanics, Asians, and Native

Recognizing and Managing Hyperglycemia, Ketoacidosis, and Hyperosmolar State

Hyperglycemia (high blood glucose) should not be ignored, since it may lead to immediate or long-term complications. Immediate complications include diabetic ketoacidosis in people with type 1 diabetes or hyperosmolar nonketotic state in those with type 2 diabetes. For people with known diabetes, the best way to prevent these conditions is daily self-monitoring of blood glucose levels, especially during periods of stress or illness—when the risk is greatest. In addition, regular testing can help uncover chronic hyperglycemia—for example, consistent blood glucose readings over 180 to 200 mg/dL—which may cause long-term complications. You may need to start taking oral diabetes drugs or insulin or increase your current dosage.

Listed below are the warning signs of hyperglycemia and its complications, and the appropriate steps to take if these symptoms appear. In addition, it is essential to carry medical identification and inform friends and coworkers of what to do in case of an emergency.

Hyperglycemia	Ketoacidosis	Hyperosmolar State
Symptoms • Thirst • Fatigue • Blurred vision • Frequent urination • Persistent infection	**Symptoms** • Nausea, vomiting, lack of appetite, or stomach pains • Dry or flushed skin • Fruity odor on breath • Labored breathing • Incoordination, confusion, sleepiness, or coma	**Symptoms** • Dry or parched mouth • Increased hunger, nausea, vomiting, or abdominal pain • Rapid, shallow breathing • Warm, dry skin with no sweating • Sleepiness or confusion
What To Do • Drink plenty of water. • Consult your doctor. People who control their diabetes through exercise and diet alone may need to start taking diabetes pills or insulin. Those who already take pills or insulin may need a higher dose. • After your treatment regimen has been adjusted, continue to test blood glucose regularly. Call the doctor if glucose remains high.	**What To Do** • Drink plenty of water. • Check blood glucose levels. • If blood glucose levels exceed 250 mg/dL, check urine for ketones. Call your doctor in the event of a positive ketone test—which may indicate an emergency. You will probably need to take extra insulin if ketone levels are very high. • If ketones remain high after taking extra insulin or you are vomiting uncontrollably, go to the hospital at once. • If a change in mental status occurs, an ambulance must be called at once. • Never exercise if ketone levels are high.	**What To Do** • Drink plenty of water. • Check blood glucose levels. • If blood glucose levels exceed 250 mg/dL, check urine for ketones. • Although people with type 2 diabetes rarely produce excessive ketones, blood glucose levels can soar to 1,000 mg/dL or higher. Call your physician if you have a blood glucose reading over 350 mg/dL, and go to the hospital immediately if blood glucose exceeds 500 mg/dL. • If a change in mental status occurs, an ambulance must be called at once.

Americans); have had a baby weighing more than 9 lbs. or were diagnosed with diabetes during pregnancy; or have high blood pressure (140/90 mm Hg or higher), low levels of high density lipoprotein cholesterol (less than 40 mg/dL), high triglyceride levels (150 mg/dL or higher), or pre-diabetes. If diabetes is diagnosed, the progression of the disease is monitored through regular laboratory tests and physical examinations.

Laboratory Tests

Pre-diabetes and diabetes are diagnosed by measuring blood glucose levels with a fasting blood glucose test or oral glucose tolerance test. If diabetes is diagnosed, a hemoglobin A1c (HbA1c) test is performed periodically to monitor blood glucose control.

Fasting blood glucose test. This test measures blood glucose levels after an overnight fast. A diagnosis of diabetes is made when the fasting blood glucose level is above 125 mg/dL on at least two tests. Fasting blood glucose values between 110 and 125 mg/dL indicate pre-diabetes. A normal fasting blood glucose level is less than 110 mg/dL.

Oral glucose tolerance test. An oral glucose tolerance test may be used to diagnose diabetes, but it is not necessary if a fasting blood glucose test indicates the presence of diabetes. In this test, an individual ingests a drink containing 75 g of glucose after an overnight fast. A diagnosis of diabetes is made if two hours later the blood glucose level is 200 mg/dL or more. Pre-diabetes is diagnosed if the two-hour blood glucose levels are between 140 and 199 mg/dL. Normal glucose levels are less than 140 mg/dL at two hours.

Hemoglobin A1c test. The HbA1c test is used in people already diagnosed with diabetes. It measures the amount of glucose attached to hemoglobin—the oxygen-carrying protein in red blood cells that gives blood its color. As blood glucose levels rise, so does the amount of glucose attached to hemoglobin. Since hemoglobin circulates in the blood until the red blood cells die (half the red blood cells are replaced every 120 days), the HbA1c test is useful for measuring average blood glucose levels over the past two to three months. People with diabetes should have a HbA1c test every three to six months; they should aim to keep their HbA1c levels below 7%.

Other laboratory tests. In addition to measures of blood glucose and HbA1c, initial and subsequent doctor visits may include tests of blood urea nitrogen (BUN), blood creatinine, and protein (albumin) in the urine to check for kidney damage, as well as measurements of

Goals for Diabetes Tests

Diabetes increases the risk of heart attacks, strokes, and problems with the eyes, kidneys, and nerves. Because keeping blood glucose, blood pressure, and blood lipids under control can reduce the risk of these complications, your doctor will periodically perform certain tests to see how well you are managing your diabetes and whether complications are developing. The table below shows the goals for some of these tests for people with diabetes. If you have not reached these goals, talk to your doctor. You may need to make some changes in your treatment regimen.

Test	Goal
Blood pressure	<130/80 mm Hg
Hemoglobin A1c	<7%
Fasting blood glucose	90–130 mg/dL
Low density lipoprotein (LDL) cholesterol	<100 mg/dL
High density lipoprotein (HDL) cholesterol	Men: >45 mg/dL Women: >55 mg/dL
Fasting triglycerides	<150 mg/dL
Urine microalbumin (random, spot test)	<30 mcg albumin/mg creatine

blood triglycerides, total cholesterol, low density lipoprotein (LDL, or "bad") cholesterol, and high density lipoprotein (HDL, or "good") cholesterol to assess risk factors for CHD.

Medical History and Physical Examination

The medical history should cover the time and circumstances of the diabetes diagnosis; dietary habits; weight history; use of oral diabetes drugs; insulin use, including the amount and time of administration; symptoms of long-term diabetes complications; effectiveness of blood glucose control (symptoms of high blood glucose and blood glucose values); frequency and timing of symptoms of hypoglycemia (low blood glucose); history of diabetic ketoacidosis; alcohol and tobacco use; exercise habits; family history of diabetes, CHD, and stroke; and other medications taken.

A physical examination should include measurements of weight and blood pressure; a dilated eye examination (performed by an ophthalmologist, a medical doctor who specializes in diseases of the eye); and a foot inspection to look for problems such as ulcers and other skin abnormalities, joint problems, and loss of sensation.

LONG-TERM COMPLICATIONS OF DIABETES

Many of the chronic, or long-term, complications of type 1 and type 2 diabetes are directly related to elevated blood glucose levels. Long-term complications include microvascular disease (abnormalities of small blood vessels), neuropathy (nerve damage), changes to the eyes, skin, gums, and teeth, and macrovascular disease (abnormalities of large blood vessels). The complications typically appear only after years or decades of having the disease, and their development is not inevitable.

Strong evidence exists that good control of blood glucose and other risk factors, such as high blood pressure, can prevent or delay the onset of long-term complications and may reduce their severity if they occur. However, improved glucose control may not reverse these complications once they appear. Treatments for long-term complications of diabetes are covered on pages 46–54.

Microvascular Disease

Microvascular disease due to diabetes affects the eyes and kidneys.

Retinopathy. Diabetic retinopathy, which affects more than 5.3 million Americans, is the most common eye complication of diabetes. Almost all people with type 1 diabetes and more than 70% with type 2 disease eventually develop retinopathy, in most cases without experiencing any vision loss.

Retinopathy is characterized by damage to the retina, the light-sensitive nerve tissue at the back of the eye that transmits visual images to the brain. This damage is caused by changes in the tiny blood vessels that supply the retina. In its early stages—called nonproliferative retinopathy—the retinal blood vessels weaken and develop bulges that may leak blood or fluid into the surrounding tissue. Vision is rarely affected during this stage.

Later on, however, patients can develop proliferative retinopathy. At this stage, fragile new blood vessels begin to grow on the retina and into the vitreous humor (the jellylike substance inside the back of eye). These abnormal blood vessels are prone to rupture and bleed into the vitreous humor, causing blurred vision or temporary blindness. Scar tissue resulting from the bleeding can pull the retina away from the back of the eye (a condition called retinal detachment) and lead to permanent vision loss.

At any stage of retinopathy, severe blurring of vision may occur if fluid accumulates around the macula. The macula is the most sensitive portion of the retina and is crucial for seeing fine detail.

NEW RESEARCH

Body Fat Location May Affect Diabetes Risk in Older Adults

The risk of type 2 diabetes is highest in people over age 65, yet this age group has a lower prevalence of obesity than people in their 50s. Obesity is a risk factor for diabetes, but in older adults the increased risk may be a result of where the fat is located, rather than the total amount of body fat, according to a recent study.

Researchers measured the height and weight of nearly 3,000 men and women (average age 74) and used computed tomography (CT) scans to measure the fat in their abdomen and thighs. Although obese men and women (those with a body mass index [BMI] of 30 or more) had the highest rate of type 2 diabetes (39% and 34%, respectively), 68% of the men and 52% of the women with type 2 diabetes were not obese. In fact, 22% of normal-weight men (BMI of less than 25) and 12% of normal-weight women had type 2 diabetes.

Participants with more abdominal and thigh fat, regardless of their BMI, were at higher risk for type 2 diabetes than those with less fat in these locations.

The researchers conclude that obesity is not as strongly linked to type 2 diabetes in older adults as it is in younger people. Instead, excess fat in locations such as the abdomen or thighs might be a more powerful predictor of diabetes risk in this age group.

DIABETES CARE
Volume 26, page 372
February 2003

This condition is called macular edema. If detected early, both macular edema and proliferative retinopathy can be treated with a procedure called laser photocoagulation (see the feature on page 47). Prompt treatment can also spare vision in those with retinal detachment.

The most important way to prevent diabetic retinopathy or keep it from getting worse is to maintain blood glucose levels as close to normal as possible. In the Diabetes Control and Complications Trial (DCCT; see pages 21–22), people with type 1 diabetes who gave themselves multiple insulin injections each day or used an insulin pump reduced their risk of developing diabetic retinopathy by 76% and lowered their risk of having existing retinopathy progress by 54%, compared with people who followed a less rigorous treatment program. In addition, the United Kingdom Prospective Diabetes Study (UKPDS; see pages 21–22) found that people with type 2 diabetes who controlled their blood glucose levels with medication were 30% less likely to have retinopathy that required laser treatment than people who relied on diet and exercise alone.

An annual dilated eye examination performed by an ophthalmologist is also essential to detect diabetic retinopathy in its early stages and monitor its progression. In addition, lowering blood pressure below 130/80 mm Hg can help prevent the onset and progression of damage to the retina. Some—but not all—studies indicate that lowering blood cholesterol levels and quitting smoking may be helpful as well.

Nephropathy. About 30% to 40% of people with type 1 diabetes and 20% of those with type 2 diabetes develop kidney damage (nephropathy) that can lead to kidney failure, as well as to an increased risk of heart attack and stroke. The DCCT showed that intensive diabetes management in people with type 1 diabetes can reduce the risk of kidney damage by 50%.

The first detectable sign of nephropathy is the appearance of small amounts of a protein called albumin in the urine (microalbuminuria). Microalbuminuria usually develops after 10 to 15 years of diabetes. Over the next 8 to 10 years, progression of kidney damage may cause leakage of large amounts of protein in the urine (proteinuria), accumulation of waste products in the blood (azotemia), and—finally—kidney failure, which requires treatment with dialysis or a kidney transplant.

To detect kidney damage in its early stages, people with diabetes should have a urine microalbumin test once a year.

NEW RESEARCH

Watching TV Linked to Obesity, Diabetes

People who watch large amounts of television increase their risk of becoming obese and developing diabetes, regardless of how much they exercise.

Doctors from Harvard found that every two hours a day spent watching television increased the risk of obesity by 23% and diabetes by 14%, independent of exercise levels. However, for every two hours a day spent walking or standing at home during activities like housework, the risks decreased by 9% for obesity and by 12% for diabetes.

The study involved data from 68,497 women who were followed for six years while participating in the Nurses' Health Study.

The authors of the report conclude that watching fewer than 10 hours of television per week and walking briskly for 30 or more minutes per day could prevent 30% and 43% of new cases of obesity and type 2 diabetes, respectively.

Television watching may lead to obesity, and therefore diabetes, because people tend to eat more food (especially unhealthy foods) while watching television than during other sedentary activities.

JOURNAL OF THE AMERICAN MEDICAL ASSOCIATION
Volume 289, page 1785
April 9, 2003

How To Deal With Skin Problems

If you have diabetes, it's critical to take good care of your skin.

Diabetes can have some surprising effects on the largest organ in your body—the skin. In fact, about 30% of people with diabetes experience a diabetes-related skin problem at some point. Not all of these skin problems result from poor blood glucose control; some crop up even in people with well-controlled diabetes. While some diabetes-related skin problems require no treatment at all or can be cared for at home, others can be serious and require medical attention.

If you have diabetes, you should become familiar with the common skin problems related to the condition and learn good day-to-day skin-care techniques to prevent many of these problems.

Fungal Infection

What is it? In people with diabetes, fungal infections are common and occur in several varieties. Most common are vaginal yeast infections in women with uncontrolled diabetes. Fungal infections of the toenails (onychomycosis) can occur as well. In people with poorly controlled diabetes, fungal infections can also occur as itchy red patches of skin encircled by small scales and blisters in areas where skin rubs against skin, such as the armpits, groin, and between the toes.

How is it treated? The two main treatments for fungal infections are good blood glucose control and topical antifungal medications.

Acanthosis Nigricans

What is it? Acanthosis nigricans is characterized by velvety, soft areas of darkened skin. It usually appears on the neck or armpits but is sometimes found on the hands, knees, or elbows. The condition is more common in blacks, Hispanics, and Native Americans than in whites. It is a sign of insulin resistance, meaning that your pancreas is working overtime or that you may need higher doses of insulin if you are on insulin therapy. Acanthosis nigricans can also occur in people with pre-diabetes.

How is it treated? Acanthosis nigricans doesn't require treatment.

Diabetic Dermopathy

What is it? Sometimes called shin spots, diabetic dermopathy is the most common skin condition in people with diabetes. It appears as reddish-brown, scaly spots that are round or oval and usually occur on the shins but also sometimes on the forearms, feet, or thighs. The spots can eventually develop into shallow, dark scars. Diabetic dermopathy may be the result of damage to the skin (usually from heat, cold, or bumping something) or just the slow healing of abrasions.

How is it treated? Diabetic dermopathy does not need to be treated since it doesn't progress into a more serious condition.

Necrobiosis Lipoidica Diabeticorum

What is it? Necrobiosis lipoidica diabeticorum is a rare condition, occurring in only 0.3% of people with diabetes each year. It is most common in women in their 20s or 30s and is characterized by reddish-purple, round lesions. The lesions are usually on the lower leg, ankle, or feet but can also occur on the scalp, face, forearms, hands, or abdomen. They start small but can enlarge to as much as an inch or more in diameter. Over time, the lesions often become transparent, and the blood vessels below can be seen. Rarely, the spots become painful and itchy.

How is it treated? Up to 19% of cases of necrobiosis lipoidica diabeticorum become inactive on their own over the years (that is, they become stable dark or purple spots). Treatment is not required unless the lesions ulcerate (open), which happens occasionally. If ulceration occurs, your doctor may prescribe topical corticosteroids. Blood glucose control does not appear to affect the risk or progression of this condition.

Granuloma Annulare

What is it? Granuloma annulare appears as ring- or arc-shaped, raised lesions that are red, reddish-brown, or

Neuropathy

About 60% to 70% of people with diabetes develop nerve damage (neuropathy), though they may experience no symptoms. Neuropathy typically develops slowly. The best way to prevent it is to maintain good control of blood glucose. According to the DCCT, tight control of blood glucose can decrease the risk of neuropathy by 60%.

flesh colored. Usually the condition occurs symmetrically on the ears, fingers, neck, arms, legs, or trunk.

How is it treated? Topical corticosteroids may be of use. The exact role of blood glucose levels in the condition is unknown.

Eruptive Xanthomatosis

What is it? Eruptive xanthomatosis is characterized by yellow pimples surrounded by red edges. The pimples generally occur on the elbows, hands, arms, legs, trunk, back, or buttocks and are the result of extremely high blood triglyceride levels—greater than 1,000 mg/dL. The condition can cause itching. It is most common in young males with type 1 diabetes.

How is it treated? Eruptive xanthomatosis goes away once triglyceride levels are brought under control. Medications to lower triglyceride levels are often required because such very high levels of triglycerides can also cause pancreatitis (inflammation of the pancreas).

Bacterial Infection

What is it? Bacterial infections result in skin that is painful, red, hot, and swollen. In people with diabetes, bacterial infections of the skin often appear as boils (infections of the hair follicles), carbuncles (groups of boils), or styes (infections of the eyelash follicles). Bacterial infections also can form in the skin surrounding the nails.

How is it treated? These infections can be managed through good blood glucose control, antibiotics, and, if necessary, removal of the affected tissue by a doctor.

Bullosis Diabeticorum

What is it? Also known as diabetic blisters, bullosis diabeticorum is a rare condition that occurs almost exclusively in people with diabetes. It appears as painless blisters that contain a clear fluid. The blisters usually occur on the toes and feet but sometimes on the legs, forearms, fingers, and hands.

How is it treated? Some diabetic blisters heal on their own within about five weeks and do not scar; others result in scarring. The only way to treat this condition is to control blood glucose levels. Also, take care to avoid having the blisters burst and to prevent infections if they do burst.

14 Skin Care Tips

Because diabetes puts you at increased risk for many skin conditions, it is important that you take extra precautions:

- Control your blood glucose levels.
- Drink plenty of fluids—this helps prevent dry skin.
- Treat cuts quickly. Wash them with water and mild soap, dry them carefully (being sure not to make the opening worse), apply antibiotic ointment if your doctor recommends it, and cover with sterile gauze. See your doctor if the cut is large.
- Use warm (not hot) water in the bath or shower.
- Try not to bathe frequently, especially when the humidity is low. Otherwise, your skin can become dry.
- Use a mild soap (preferably one with moisturizer, such as Basis or Dove), and be sure to rinse off the soap completely.
- Don't take bubble baths if you have dry skin.
- Dry yourself thoroughly after bathing, and check for any unusual patches, blemishes, or lesions on your skin.
- Use moisturizer after you bathe. Lubriderm and Alpha Keri are good options. Avoid putting any moisturizer between your toes.
- Place cornstarch in places where moisture can accumulate, like the armpits, groin, and between the toes.
- Don't scratch itchy skin. This can cause it to open up, increasing the risk of an infection. Instead, use moisturizer.
- Wear underwear made of cotton rather than synthetic fabric, because cotton "breathes" better.
- Use a humidifier in your home, especially during dry times of the year.
- Consult your doctor about any skin problem that doesn't get better on its own or that you cannot treat with self-care measures.

Diabetes can cause three types of neuropathy: peripheral neuropathy, mononeuropathy, and autonomic neuropathy. The most common type is peripheral neuropathy; it involves a slow, progressive loss of function of the sensory nerves in the limbs. Symptoms include numbness, tingling, and pain in the legs and hands on both sides of the body. The nerve damage responds to improved blood glucose control slowly, if at all.

Mononeuropathy results from a disruption of the blood supply to a single nerve or nerve group. It leads to sudden pain or weakness in the area of the body served by the affected nerve or nerve group. Symptoms gradually improve over two to six months without any treatment.

Autonomic neuropathy develops when diabetes damages the autonomic nervous system, which regulates bodily functions that are not under voluntary control—for example, digestion, heart rate, and blood pressure. Symptoms of autonomic neuropathy include stomach, bowel, or bladder problems, sexual dysfunction, dizziness, rapid or irregular heartbeat, and abnormal sweating. Most people with autonomic neuropathy also have significant peripheral neuropathy.

Cataracts and Glaucoma

Cataracts and glaucoma are eye diseases that occur with increased frequency in people with diabetes. Cataracts cause clouding of the lens of the eye; glaucoma results in damage to the optic nerve, which carries visual information from the retina to the brain. Elevated levels of sorbitol, a sugar formed from glucose, within the lens of the eye may enhance cataract formation in people with diabetes. Cataracts are usually treated only when they begin to interfere with vision. Regular testing for glaucoma is essential, since serious damage may occur before it causes symptoms.

Skin Changes

People with diabetes are at increased risk for a number of skin conditions, some of which occur despite good blood glucose control. Diabetic dermopathy is the most common diabetes-related skin problem. Also called shin spots, diabetic dermopathy appears as reddish-brown, scaly lesions about half an inch in diameter. People with diabetes also are more susceptible to skin infections. Unlike shin spots, which are harmless and require no treatment, infections can be serious and require medical attention. For more information on skin conditions that can affect people with diabetes, and how to prevent and treat them, see the feature on pages 14–15.

Dental Changes

Diabetes can lead to complications of the teeth and gums, as well as to dry mouth. Because saliva protects against bacterial growth in the mouth, and insufficient saliva permits dental plaque and food particles to accumulate, people with poorly controlled diabetes are more likely to develop cavities. As a result of excess plaque formation, two gum disorders—gingivitis and the more serious periodontitis—also are more common in people with diabetes. However, the risk of cavities can be minimized by avoiding foods high in sugar (such as candy and soda) and by carefully following an oral health regimen. A burning sensation in the mouth or on the tongue can result from dry mouth or diabetic neuropathy.

Macrovascular Disease

People with diabetes are highly susceptible to atherosclerosis—the buildup of deposits called plaques in arteries. These plaques narrow the arteries and can lead to heart attacks, strokes, or peripheral vascular disease (poor blood flow to the legs). These complications are the cause of death in three quarters of people with diabetes.

Metabolic syndrome. Elevated blood glucose levels, high blood pressure, abdominal obesity, high blood triglyceride levels, and low HDL cholesterol levels occur together in some people. This cluster of symptoms is known as metabolic syndrome. Nearly 25% of Americans have metabolic syndrome, and the condition increases their risk of diabetes, CHD, and stroke. The symptoms and risks of metabolic syndrome can be avoided by controlling body weight (preferably through a combination of diet and exercise), blood pressure, and blood lipids (cholesterol and triglycerides) and by quitting smoking. For more information on metabolic syndrome, see the feature on pages 18–19.

Coronary heart disease (CHD). People with diabetes have a two to four times greater likelihood of developing CHD than people without diabetes. CHD occurs when the coronary arteries (arteries that carry blood to the heart) become narrowed by atherosclerosis. Partial blockage of the coronary arteries produces angina (chest pain); complete blockage results in a heart attack.

The Framingham Heart Study and many others have shown that diabetes adds significantly to conventional CHD risk factors like smoking, high blood pressure, elevated LDL cholesterol, and low HDL cholesterol. In fact, a Finnish study recently found that people with type 2 diabetes who have no history of CHD have the same risk of a heart attack as those without diabetes who have already had a heart attack.

To reduce the risk of CHD, people with diabetes need to control the ABCs of diabetes: Hb**A**1c, **b**lood pressure, and **c**holesterol. The goal is to achieve an HbA1c level below 7%, a blood pressure less than 130/80 mm Hg, and an LDL cholesterol level lower than

NEW RESEARCH

Metabolic Syndrome Increases Risk of Heart Attack, Diabetes

Men with metabolic syndrome have a significantly elevated risk of having a heart attack or developing diabetes, according to a study of Scottish men.

Researchers identified the presence of metabolic syndrome and measured blood levels of C-reactive protein (CRP; a marker for inflammation) in 6,447 men with moderately high levels of low density lipoprotein (LDL) cholesterol who had never had a heart attack or diabetes. Men were considered to have metabolic syndrome if they had at least three of these factors: high triglycerides, high blood pressure, low high density lipoprotein (HDL) cholesterol, elevated fasting blood glucose, or obesity.

After nearly five years, men who had metabolic syndrome were almost two times more likely as men without metabolic syndrome to have had a nonfatal heart attack or to have died of coronary heart disease (CHD); they also had a 3½-fold increased risk of diabetes. The presence of four or five risk factors for metabolic syndrome was associated with a significant increase in risk, as were CRP levels above 3 mg/L.

Using these five factors to diagnose people with metabolic syndrome "will help identify individuals who may receive particular benefit from lifestyle measures to prevent CHD and diabetes," the researchers conclude.

CIRCULATION
Volume 108, page 414
July 29, 2003

Metabolic Syndrome: A Cluster of Related Problems

Most people have never heard of this surprisingly common condition in which insulin resistance plays a key role.

For many years, physicians have recognized that elevated blood glucose levels, high blood pressure, obesity, and abnormal blood lipid levels tend to occur together in certain individuals. This cluster of symptoms—previously called "The Deadly Quartet," syndrome X, or insulin resistance syndrome—is now commonly referred to as metabolic syndrome. Almost one in four American adults has metabolic syndrome, which increases the risk of diabetes, coronary heart disease, and stroke.

Diagnosis and Prevalence

In 2001, the National Cholesterol Education Program (sponsored by the National Heart, Lung, and Blood Institute) proposed the following criteria for the diagnosis of metabolic syndrome. A person needs to have at least three of the following five factors to be diagnosed with the condition:

- abdominal obesity (a waist circumference greater than 40 inches in men or 35 inches in women);
- triglyceride levels of 150 mg/dL or greater;
- high density lipoprotein (HDL) cholesterol levels of less than 40 mg/dL in men or 50 mg/dL in women;
- blood pressures of 130/85 mm Hg or higher, or taking antihypertensive medication; and
- fasting blood glucose levels of 110 mg/dL or greater.

While only 7% of men and women age 20 to 29 meet this definition of metabolic syndrome, the percentage rises to more than 40% of those age 60 and older. The condition is more common in Mexican Americans (32%) than in whites (24%) or blacks (22%).

Causes

Virtually all people with metabolic syndrome have insulin resistance, a decreased ability of the body's tissues to respond to insulin. Insulin enables cells to take up glucose from the blood for use as a source of energy. In people with insulin resistance, the cells don't respond adequately to the effects of insulin, and insufficient amounts of glucose enter the cells. As a result, the pancreas produces more insulin to help move glucose into the cells, and blood insulin levels rise. Eventually, the pancreas can no longer produce enough insulin to compensate for the insulin resistance, blood glucose levels rise, and diabetes develops.

Even before the onset of diabetes, however, people may have elevated blood pressure. Increased production of triglycerides by the liver can lead to abnormalities in blood lipid levels, including high triglycerides, low levels of HDL cholesterol, and increased levels of small, dense low density lipoprotein (LDL), which is more likely to cause blood clots than less-dense LDL.

Exactly what causes insulin resistance is unclear. However, researchers do know that genetic factors, obesity, physical inactivity, diet, cigarette smoking, and older age each contribute to insulin resistance and therefore to metabolic syndrome. Other factors that make a person more likely to develop insulin resistance include a family history of diabetes in a first-degree relative (a parent or sibling), a personal history of gestational diabetes (diabetes during pregnancy), or polycystic ovary syndrome (a

100 mg/dL. Some people can achieve these goals through diet and exercise alone, while others will require medication. Quitting smoking and taking an aspirin daily also can reduce the risk of CHD, as can keeping triglyceride levels below 150 mg/dL and HDL cholesterol levels higher than 45 mg/dL in men and 55 mg/dL in women.

Stroke. People with diabetes are two to four times more likely to suffer a stroke than those without diabetes. A stroke occurs when a clot blocks blood flow through an artery that leads to the brain. Experts suspect that high blood glucose increases the risk of stroke by promoting atherosclerosis and clots. In addition, high blood pressure—one of the most important risk factors for stroke—is twice as common in people with diabetes than those without the disease.

As is the case for CHD prevention, controlling the ABCs of diabetes is critical to reducing the risk of stroke. Levels of HbA1c condition characterized by infrequent or absent menstruation, infertility, and excessive body hair).

Complications

Metabolic syndrome increases the risk of numerous complications. Because of its association with insulin resistance, people with metabolic syndrome are more likely to have type 2 diabetes. In turn, diabetes increases the risk of vision problems, kidney dysfunction, nerve problems, coronary heart disease, and stroke.

High blood pressure, high triglyceride levels, and low HDL cholesterol levels are all risk factors for atherosclerosis. Elevated insulin levels are also associated with an increased tendency for blood to clot. As a result, people with metabolic syndrome have a greater incidence of all types of cardiovascular disease (including nonfatal and fatal heart attacks and strokes) and are at increased risk for premature death from any cause.

Treatment

Treatment of metabolic syndrome focuses on overcoming insulin resistance and correcting any associated abnormalities. The first step in treatment is lifestyle changes. The most important lifestyle change is weight loss through increased physical activity, decreased intake of calories (particularly simple carbohydrates), and increased fiber intake.

Physical activity aids in weight loss, improves responsiveness to insulin, increases HDL cholesterol levels, and decreases blood pressure. An increase in activity need not be dramatic to achieve significant health benefits—even a half hour of brisk walking most days of the week will help.

Weight loss improves insulin sensitivity, reduces elevated insulin levels, and lowers the risk of developing type 2 diabetes. While reduced insulin resistance can occur with as little as a 5-lb. weight loss, better results are achieved with a 7% to 15% decrease in body weight.

A diet rich in fiber-containing foods—such as fruits, vegetables, and whole grains—can help overcome insulin resistance. Smoking cessation can lessen insulin resistance and help to raise HDL cholesterol levels.

If lifestyle modifications do not correct the associated cardiovascular risk factors, medications can lower blood pressure and improve lipid levels. Thiazide diuretics are considered first-choice therapy for high blood pressure because they also prevent heart attacks and strokes. In addition, ACE inhibitors are a good choice for those with metabolic syndrome because they may reduce the risk of type 2 diabetes in addition to lowering blood pressure. Some people with metabolic syndrome may require statins, which lower LDL cholesterol and raise HDL cholesterol levels. Niacin, gemfibrozil (Lopid), and fenofibrate (Lofibra, Tricor) can also raise HDL cholesterol and lower triglyceride levels.

Metformin (Glucophage) and the thiazolidinediones pioglitazone (Actos) and rosiglitazone (Avandia) are currently used to treat insulin resistance in people with type 2 diabetes. According to a 2002 study in *The New England Journal of Medicine,* people at high risk for diabetes (those who are overweight and have elevated blood glucose levels) can prevent or delay the development of diabetes with lifestyle changes and, less markedly, with metformin. However, it is not yet clear whether these medications should be used to treat the insulin resistance that leads to metabolic syndrome.

should be below 7%; blood pressure less than 130/80 mm Hg; and LDL cholesterol levels lower than 100 mg/dL. Quitting smoking and taking an aspirin daily may be beneficial as well.

Peripheral vascular disease. Peripheral vascular disease is a narrowing of the arteries in the legs due to atherosclerosis. The characteristic symptom of the condition is intermittent claudication—pain in the thighs, calves, and, sometimes, the buttocks—that is brought on by exercise and subsides promptly with rest. In most people, pain occurs after a predictable amount of physical activity.

Symptoms of peripheral vascular disease usually progress slowly. Eventually the pain can interfere with normal activities and may even occur at rest if blood vessels are severely narrowed. The poor blood flow in the legs can result in slow healing of foot blisters and other skin injuries and may lead to chronic ulcers on the feet and legs.

Diabetes doubles the risk of peripheral vascular disease. Preventive measures are the same as those for CHD and stroke: HbA1c levels less than 7%, blood pressure below 130/80 mm Hg, and LDL cholesterol levels lower than 100 mg/dL.

Diabetic Foot Problems

People with diabetes need to pay special attention to their feet for a number of reasons. Diabetes-related nerve damage can reduce feeling in the feet, making it difficult to detect a foot injury. Diabetes can also impair blood circulation and wound healing by narrowing the arteries supplying blood to the legs. A wound on the foot that does not heal can turn into an ulcer (deep sore) that may become infected and possibly even require an amputation if untreated. The risk of these complications can be reduced by keeping diabetes well controlled, having a foot inspection performed by a family doctor or podiatrist at least twice a year, and taking care of the feet as described on pages 50–52.

TREATMENT OF DIABETES

The goals in the treatment of diabetes are to prevent its acute manifestations (hyperglycemia, hypoglycemia, diabetic ketoacidosis, and hyperosmolar nonketotic state) and its long-term complications (such as retinopathy, nephropathy, neuropathy, and macrovascular disease). Eating a healthy diet and exercising regularly are the first steps in treating diabetes, but some form of drug treatment is often needed as well.

The Diabetes Health Care Team

Because even basic health care is more complicated in people with diabetes, the disorder is best treated by a team of professionals who have specialized knowledge about the disease. Members of the health care team who have the initials *C.D.E.* after their name have passed a special certification exam on diabetes education; C.D.E. stands for certified diabetes educator. The American Diabetes Association can provide the names of certified diabetes educators in your area. (See page 58 for contact information.)

Key members of the diabetes health care team include diabetes nurse educators (registered nurses who specialize in providing instruction and advice on issues related to the day-to-day management of diabetes), diabetes specialists (medical doctors such as diabetologists and endocrinologists), primary care physicians, registered dietitians, exercise physiologists (to help people with diabetes create an individualized exercise program), mental health professionals, ophthalmologists, and podiatrists.

Tight Glucose Control

Control of blood glucose levels clearly prevents the symptoms of high blood glucose. Although doctors long suspected that meticulous blood glucose control would slow or prevent the development of microvascular complications (retinopathy and nephropathy) and neuropathy, strong evidence for this assumption only became available about a decade ago, with the results of the DCCT, a 10-year study involving 1,441 men and women with type 1 diabetes.

Participants in the DCCT followed one of two treatment regimens. People in the intensive-treatment group monitored their blood glucose levels three or four times a day, injected insulin three or four times a day (or used an insulin pump), adjusted their insulin doses according to blood glucose levels, and followed dietary and exercise recommendations daily. People in the standard-treatment group engaged in daily blood glucose monitoring, injected insulin once or twice a day, and followed standard diet and exercise recommendations.

During the study, those in the intensive-treatment group had significantly lower fasting blood glucose and HbA1c levels than those in the standard-treatment group. Moreover, the intensive-treatment group reduced their risks of diabetic complications—retinopathy by 76%, nephropathy by 50%, and neuropathy by 60%.

While this study included only individuals with type 1 diabetes, the findings of the UKPDS confirmed that improved blood glucose control provides similar protection against long-term microvascular complications in people with type 2 diabetes. In the UKPDS, researchers followed 3,867 people with type 2 diabetes for 10 years. Half of the participants were randomly assigned to a conventional-treatment program of diet and exercise; the other half followed the diet and exercise program but were also treated with diabetes medication (a sulfonylurea drug, metformin, and/or insulin). Compared with diet and exercise alone, drug therapy resulted in better glucose control and a 25% reduction in retinopathy and kidney failure.

Evidence is growing that good blood glucose control may also help prevent macrovascular complications. In a follow-up study to the DCCT, people with type 1 diabetes who maintained an HbA1c of 7% during the trial had 24% less plaque in their carotid arteries six years later than those who maintained an HbA1c of 9%. Plaques in

NEW RESEARCH

Good Glycemic Control May Protect Nerves

Keeping tight control over blood glucose levels may help prevent nerve damage in people with type 1 diabetes, according to a recent study. Other studies have found that tight control protects nerves in the short term, but the new study has the longest follow-up to date.

Researchers followed 39 people with type 1 diabetes for 18 years. The participants were between 18 and 40 years old when the study began in 1982, and they had had diabetes for 7 to 23 years. They underwent periodic HbA1c tests as well as assessments of nerve function in their legs.

During the study, the average HbA1c level for all participants was 8.2%. Participants with the best blood glucose control (HbA1c levels of less than 8.4%) were less likely to lose sensation in their legs than those with an HbA1c of 8.4% or greater.

The study did not show any association between nerve damage and other factors such as high blood pressure, cholesterol, microalbuminuria (small amounts of protein in the urine), or smoking. The researchers say the results emphasize the importance of good blood glucose control, since it appears to help protect nerves even in people who have had type 1 diabetes for more than 30 years.

DIABETES CARE
Volume 26, page 2400
August 2003

the carotid arteries can lead to a stroke. In the UKPDS, every 1% reduction in HbA1c was associated with a 14% decrease in the risk of heart attacks in people with type 2 diabetes.

The accumulated evidence has led the American Diabetes Association to conclude that all people with diabetes can benefit from better control of their blood glucose levels. However, the organization points out that aggressive glucose control might not be appropriate for everyone. Participants in the intensive-treatment group of the DCCT had a threefold higher incidence of hypoglycemia than people in the standard-treatment group.

The risks of tight blood glucose control may outweigh the possible benefits in the following people: In the very elderly, the chance of living long enough to develop long-term complications may not be as great as the risk of hypoglycemia, which can lead to dizziness, fainting, and injuries due to falls. People who do not recognize their hypoglycemic reactions (hypoglycemia unawareness), either because of repeated episodes of hypoglycemia or because they are taking a beta-blocker, may also need to relax their blood glucose control. Studies show, however, that awareness of hypoglycemia can be regained by preventing episodes of significant hypoglycemia for several months.

Nevertheless, people with diabetes—whether they have type 1 or type 2—should strive for the best blood glucose control as is safely possible. No guidelines have been set for tight control, but the intensive-treatment group in the DCCT achieved an average blood glucose level of around 155 mg/dL, which is equivalent to an HbA1c level of about 7%. While tight control always involves blood glucose monitoring, it may not require insulin injections in people with type 2 diabetes: A carefully constructed program of diet, exercise, and oral drugs (if needed) may be sufficient.

Self-Monitoring of Blood Glucose Control

Currently, the best method to monitor blood glucose control is self-testing of blood glucose using a home blood glucose meter. (Testing for the presence of glucose in the urine is not considered useful.) Results from the DCCT and other studies indicate that people with diabetes should be more aggressive in their daily monitoring of blood glucose levels if they want to reduce the risk of diabetes complications. This means not only making more frequent blood glucose measurements, but also adjusting diet, exercise, and doses of insulin or oral medications according to the results.

Along with regularly measuring blood glucose levels, people with

How To Control Blood Glucose During an Illness

Getting sick can trigger rises in blood glucose levels. The following steps can help keep blood glucose levels in check and prevent complications.

People with diabetes must be especially careful when suffering from an illness like a cold or the flu. Illness not only affects your eating, sleeping, and exercise—habits closely linked to blood glucose control—it may cause the liver to make and release glucose into the bloodstream. This increase in glucose released from the liver provides extra energy to combat the stress of an illness, but in people with diabetes it can cause blood glucose to rise too high, whether you are eating or not.

At the same time, an illness decreases the sensitivity of cells to insulin and makes it more difficult for these cells to remove glucose from the bloodstream. A person without diabetes can produce extra insulin to help the additional glucose enter cells. But people with diabetes are less able to produce extra insulin or respond to it effectively. The resulting rise in blood glucose increases the risk of diabetic ketoacidosis in people with type 1 diabetes and hyperosmolar nonketotic state in those with type 2 diabetes. To prevent these serious complications, as well as to minimize fluctuations in blood glucose levels, follow these sick-day precautions.

Inform your health care professional when you become sick. This precaution is particularly important if you are unable to eat regular foods, have diarrhea or vomiting for more than six hours, or have had a fever for a couple of days that is not improving.

Follow the treatment plan for the sickness. For example, take any necessary medications, such as antibiotics for an infection, according to schedule. If you are treated by a doctor you have never seen before, make sure he or she is aware that you have diabetes.

Test blood glucose levels more often than usual. If you have type 1 diabetes, test blood glucose and urine ketone levels every four hours, even during the night. (Set an alarm clock or have someone wake you up.) If you have type 2 diabetes, testing blood glucose levels four times during the day is probably enough; if blood glucose levels exceed 250 mg/dL, test urine for ketones. Call your health care professional if blood glucose levels are consistently above 250 mg/dL and are accompanied by ketones in the urine.

Take your diabetes medication as usual, unless, of course, your health professional advises otherwise. Being sick causes blood glucose levels to rise, even if you are not eating.

If you use insulin, keep a bottle of rapid- or very rapid-acting insulin handy. You should take this precaution even if you do not take these types of insulin regularly. Use the rapid- or very rapid-acting insulin if your health professional tells you to take an extra sick-day dose or if you need to lower blood glucose levels quickly.

Watch for any symptoms of dehydration, ketoacidosis, or hyperosmolar nonketotic state. The symptoms of dehydration include dry mouth, cracked lips, and dry or flushed skin. For the symptoms of ketoacidosis and hyperosmolar nonketotic state, see the feature on page 9. Contact your health professional if any of these symptoms occur.

Prevent dehydration by drinking plenty of liquids. You should consume at least one large (8 oz.) glass of clear fluid each hour while awake. If your usual diet is not disrupted by the illness, drink water, tea, broth, or other sugar-free beverages. If you are unable to eat meals, alternate sugar-containing fluids with those that are sugar-free.

Try to consume a normal amount of carbohydrates. Eating many small portions throughout the day may help. Eat easy-to-digest foods such as gelatin, crackers, soup, and applesauce.

Rest as much as possible. If necessary, get someone—such as a family member or friend—to help care for you.

Preventing Illness In the First Place

To prevent flu and pneumonia, the American Diabetes Association strongly recommends that people over six months of age who have diabetes receive a flu vaccine once a year. The vaccine is available at doctors' offices, clinics, and pharmacies, among other places. The best time to get vaccinated is at the beginning of the flu season—between September and November. The pneumonia vaccine is also recommended for people with diabetes. If you are over age 65 and have not had a pneumonia vaccination in the past five years, you need a second one.

diabetes should keep a log of their readings. (A log book is often included with the purchase of a blood glucose meter.) This record allows more accurate tracking of blood glucose levels and can help point out sources of difficulty in controlling diabetes. In some cases, unexpected fluctuations in blood glucose readings can be traced to simple changes in routine—for example, unusually large or small meals, variations in exercise, or even psychological stress.

An even better way to evaluate results is to download the glucose readings from the meter onto a computer. Patterns often become clear when the downloaded information is displayed on a printout.

Blood glucose testing. The availability of simple and accurate blood glucose tests, which allow people with diabetes to make immediate changes in their diet and medication, has made home glucose monitoring the backbone of diabetes management. Most blood tests require only a single drop of blood, which is withdrawn by a special lancet or the meter itself. A wide variety of devices make drawing blood as painless and simple as possible. Some are spring-loaded and adjustable to give as shallow a stick as possible; others allow blood to be withdrawn from the forearm, which is less sensitive than the fingertips.

The withdrawn blood is placed on a test strip that is impregnated with an enzyme called glucose oxidase. The blood glucose level is determined by inserting the strip into the meter; a digital readout of the result appears within 15 to 45 seconds. Recommendations for the frequency of home monitoring vary from once a day or less in people with well-controlled type 2 diabetes to multiple times daily in people with type 1 disease.

Prices for meters range from about $30 to $300 and can be greatly reduced through rebates and special offers from manufacturers. Some insurance companies offer reimbursement for certain meters and test strips. For tips on buying and maintaining a home blood glucose monitor, see the feature on page 25.

Urine glucose testing. When glucose builds up to a certain level in the blood, the excess begins to "spill over" into the urine. This typically occurs at blood glucose levels exceeding 180 mg/dL, or 200 mg/dL in older adults. Testing urine for the presence of glucose provides a rough idea of glucose control; however, it is far less useful than blood glucose monitoring. To test urine for glucose, test strips are passed through the urine stream, or drops of urine are placed on them. The presence of glucose in the urine causes a color change in the strip. The color is then compared with a chart to determine roughly how much glucose is present.

Monitoring Your Blood Glucose at Home

Choosing the right glucose meter and using it effectively can help you manage your diabetes better.

Regular home monitoring of blood glucose is essential for everyone with diabetes: It can help keep blood glucose under control and reduce the risk of many long-term complications. In addition, by recording each day's results (along with the time and prior activities such as meals or exercise), problems can be spotted as they develop, patterns in blood glucose fluctuations can be identified, and problems can be fixed early on.

Most of the blood glucose meters currently on the market require a drop of blood from your finger or forearm; less invasive models are being investigated. The following tips can help you choose and maintain an accurate blood glucose meter.

How To Choose a Meter

There are many types of blood glucose meters, so ask your doctor or diabetes educator to recommend one that meets your needs. Before buying a meter, test it out to make sure you feel comfortable using it. Also, find out how easy the meter is to maintain, clean, and calibrate.

Some meters are easier to read than others. Most models display the results digitally. Audio meters, which read the results aloud, are available for people with vision problems.

Using Your Meter Effectively

Most errors in home monitoring result from poor testing techniques, rather than from defective meters. To keep your meter in good working order, follow the manufacturer's instructions for cleaning and maintenance. Make sure your test strips are fresh (don't use them after the expiration date, or if they've changed color or have been open for a long time). Also, be sure to recalibrate your meter when needed. Dirty meters, old test strips, and improper calibration can all interfere with accuracy.

It's a good idea to test your meter's accuracy at least once a month, or whenever you suspect a problem. Follow the manufacturer's instructions carefully.

Working With Your Health Care Professional

Bring your meter to each doctor's appointment and take a reading within 5 to 10 minutes of having your blood drawn. The meter results should vary by no more than 15% from the lab's measurement. Engaging in this practice will not only help to ensure that your meter is working properly, it will also allow your doctor to monitor your technique.

Blood glucose meters with data-management systems can give a more detailed picture of your blood glucose control than traditional meters. These systems, which work with a personal digital assistant (PDA), can enhance blood glucose control by electronically recording blood glucose levels as well as information about meals and exercise. Copying or downloading this data onto your doctor's computer and displaying it graphically can make it easier to understand glucose fluctuations.

While a data-management feature is helpful, it certainly is not essential; so before buying this type of meter, make sure that you really need it and understand how to use it. Also, check to see if your model is compatible with your doctor's computer. If your doctor doesn't provide this service, your local pharmacy may be able to give you a printout of your data so you can review it with your doctor.

On the Horizon

Efforts are under way to develop less invasive blood glucose meters. For example, diabetes experts say that the development of a device that continuously measures blood glucose levels—rather than at specific points in time—will be extremely helpful. The U.S. Food and Drug Administration (FDA) has approved one such monitoring system, but it requires the insertion of a sensor just under the skin and does not provide immediate feedback to the person with diabetes. Instead, the person's doctor downloads the data every one to three days. Another device displays blood glucose levels in real time, but the device lasts only 12 hours.

Eventually, researchers hope to develop a blood glucose meter that can provide continuous blood glucose readings directly from the bloodstream; however, such a device would require major surgery to implant it.

Because urine tests are positive for glucose only when the blood glucose level is over 180 to 200 mg/dL, these tests cannot detect moderate elevations in glucose levels or hypoglycemia. In addition, there is a lag in time between when the blood glucose level is excessive and when glucose is found in the urine. Thus, anyone attempting to keep their blood glucose levels within a set range using urine glucose testing would be acting on late and incomplete information. Also, urine glucose measurements can be affected by intakes of vitamin C, aspirin, and fluids. For these reasons, urine glucose testing is rarely recommended.

Ketone testing. Ketone bodies in the urine can be measured easily by placing a test strip or tablet in urine and examining it for a color change. Typically, only people with type 1 diabetes need to perform this test. A person should check for ketones if blood glucose levels are over 250 mg/dL and symptoms such as fruity breath, nausea, vomiting, or difficulties in concentration suggest ketoacidosis. If the test is strongly positive, a doctor should be called immediately.

Dietary Measures

The right diet can help keep blood glucose levels in check and help control a number of other factors, such as elevated blood lipids (total cholesterol, LDL cholesterol, and triglycerides), obesity, and high blood pressure, that can increase the risk of developing diabetes complications.

Most experts recommend that people with diabetes eat a diet high in carbohydrates and low in fat. According to this school of thought, 50% to 60% of calories should come from carbohydrates and 30% or fewer from fat. The primary goal of this diet is to keep blood lipid levels low—to reduce the risk of macrovascular disease—without adversely affecting blood glucose levels. Most people do best when they consume a similar amount of carbohydrates at each meal, rather than trying to eliminate carbohydrates, which increases the amount of fat in the diet.

For people with diabetes, as for all adults, it is important to control the intake of total calories, saturated fat, and cholesterol. Weight loss is extremely important for those who are overweight. It not only improves control of blood glucose and blood pressure but may also lower total cholesterol, raise HDL cholesterol, and reduce triglyceride levels.

The most effective way to lose weight is to combine a lower intake of calories with exercise. This combination not only produces faster and more permanent weight loss but also prevents excessive loss of muscle mass (which burns more calories even at rest) and strengthens the cardiovascular system. Approximately 1 lb. of body weight is lost for every 3,500 calories of reduced food intake or increased energy expenditure. Highly regimented diets work temporarily for many people but are usually extremely difficult to follow

NEW RESEARCH

Eating Fish May Help Prevent Heart Disease in People With Diabetes

Frequent consumption of fish containing omega-3 fatty acids is associated with a reduced risk of coronary heart disease (CHD) in women with diabetes, according to a recent study. As a result, people with diabetes may benefit from eating at least two servings per week of fatty fish such as mackerel, herring, sardines, albacore tuna, and salmon.

More than 5,100 women with type 2 diabetes answered questions about their diet and health status every two years from 1976 to 1994. After adjusting for age and other risk factors for CHD, women who ate fish less than once a month had the highest risk of CHD. Compared with these women, CHD was 30% less likely in women who ate fish one to three times per month, 40% less likely in those who ate fish once a week, and 64% less likely in those who ate fish five or more times per week.

Nevertheless, it is unclear whether eating fish was responsible for the decrease in heart disease. Omega-3 fatty acids may protect against CHD by lowering triglyceride levels, reducing blood clot formation, and preventing irregular heart rhythms. The study authors say concerns have been raised that fish oil may interfere with blood glucose control, but two recent meta-analyses found that it does not.

CIRCULATION
Volume 107, page 1852
April 15, 2003

over the long term. Ultimately, such rigid diets need to be transformed into more balanced, healthy, and sustainable dietary habits.

Saturated fat raises blood cholesterol levels and should make up no more than 10% of total calories. To lower LDL cholesterol levels to the goal of less than 100 mg/dL, people with diabetes may need to restrict their intake of saturated fat to less than 7% of total calories. Some studies have found that saturated fat may also elevate blood insulin levels, which could contribute to CHD. In one study of about 650 men without diabetes, reducing saturated fat intake from 14% to 8% of total calories lowered fasting insulin levels by 18% and postmeal insulin levels by 25%.

Although dietary cholesterol has a smaller impact on blood lipid levels than saturated fat, people with diabetes should still limit their intake to no more than 300 mg each day. If LDL cholesterol is not at the goal of less than 100 mg/dL, cholesterol intake should not exceed 200 mg per day.

Rather than calculating the percent of calories from saturated fat and counting milligrams of cholesterol, it may be easier to simply cut back on foods high in these substances. Foods high in saturated fat include red meats, dark meat poultry, poultry skin, whole-milk dairy products, butter, and products made with hydrogenated oils or coconut, palm, or palm kernel oils. Cholesterol is found only in animal products and is particularly plentiful in egg yolks, organ meats, shrimp, crab, and lobster.

Another way to reduce saturated fat in the diet is to replace it with monounsaturated fat. Monounsaturated fat—which is plentiful in olive oil, canola oil, avocados, and some nuts—lowers total blood cholesterol levels without reducing HDL cholesterol. (Polyunsaturated fat found in vegetable oils like safflower, corn, sunflower, and soybean oils lowers total cholesterol levels but may also reduce HDL cholesterol.) Furthermore, the substitution of monounsaturated fat for polyunsaturated fat in the diet decreases the likelihood of LDL oxidation, which is thought to initiate the accumulation of LDL cholesterol in the walls of arteries—one of the first steps in the development of atherosclerosis.

Other dietary considerations for people with diabetes include the following.

Dietary fiber. Fiber is a type of carbohydrate that is not broken down in the intestine. Some studies have shown that a diet high in soluble fiber—found in oats, oat bran, legumes, barley, citrus fruits, and apples—can help lower blood glucose and blood cholesterol levels. Insoluble fiber—found in whole wheat, wheat bran, vegetables,

NEW RESEARCH

Whole-Grain Foods May Help Prevent Type 2 Diabetes

A new study finds that a diet high in fiber from whole-grain foods may help prevent type 2 diabetes in both men and women.

Researchers in Finland assessed the dietary habits of more than 2,200 men and more than 2,000 women (age 40 to 69) who did not have diabetes. Ten years later, 54 men and 102 women had developed type 2 diabetes.

When the participants were divided into four groups based on their consumption of whole-grain foods, those with the highest consumption were 35% less likely to have diabetes than those with the lowest consumption. In addition, those consuming the most fiber from cereal were 61% less likely to have developed diabetes than those consuming the least, suggesting that the association between whole grains and diabetes is largely due to cereal fiber.

The study does not prove that diets high in whole-grain foods prevent diabetes, but it suggests that people who eat these diets have some protective factors. The researchers offer two possible explanations. First, soluble fiber may slow the absorption of carbohydrates and so reduce the demand for insulin. Second, insoluble fiber moves carbohydrates more quickly through the intestines, leaving less time for the body to absorb the carbohydrates.

AMERICAN JOURNAL OF CLINICAL NUTRITION
Volume 77, pages 527 and 622
March 2003

and fruit—can help prevent constipation. Both types of fiber are needed for a healthy diet.

Experts are unsure how fiber lowers blood glucose. One theory is that fiber slows the digestion of food, delaying the breakdown of carbohydrates and the absorption of glucose into the bloodstream. The resulting smaller rise in blood glucose after meals gives insulin more of an opportunity to convert the glucose into energy. The American Diabetes Association recommends consuming 20 to 35 g of dietary fiber each day.

Sugar. The American Diabetes Association recently relaxed its restrictions on sugar (sucrose) intake for people with diabetes. This change was made because sugars (such as those in sweets and sodas) and starches (such as those in pasta, rice, and breads) affect blood glucose levels similarly when eaten in exactly the same amounts. In other words, the total amount of carbohydrates eaten is more important than the type of carbohydrates.

But the problem is that a small portion of sugar equals the carbohydrate content of a much larger serving of starch. For example, just one tablespoon of sugar contains the same amount of carbohydrates as a 3-oz. baked potato. Consequently, it is easy to ingest too many carbohydrates when eating sugary rather than starchy foods.

As long as sugar replaces other carbohydrates gram for gram (calorie for calorie) and is not simply added to the diet, it is safe for people with diabetes to consume foods that contain sugar. Remember, however, that sugary foods often contain empty calories, whereas starchy foods also supply vitamins, minerals, and fiber. Therefore, for overall health it is preferable for people with diabetes to avoid sugar-containing foods. (Artificial sweeteners approved by the FDA, such as saccharin, aspartame, acesulfame potassium, and sucralose are not restricted.)

Antioxidants. Antioxidants are chemical compounds that help prevent cell damage by inactivating molecules called free radicals that are formed during the normal course of metabolism. Some examples of antioxidants are vitamin C, vitamin E, selenium, and beta-carotene. Although population studies suggested that vitamin E might reduce the risk of macrovascular disease by protecting against LDL oxidation, in three large trials, vitamin E supplements did not prevent heart attacks and strokes in people with known CHD or in people with diabetes and other CHD risk factors.

Sodium. People with diabetes and high blood pressure should restrict their sodium intake to less than 2,500 mg per day to help lower their blood pressure. This level of sodium restriction can be

The Truth About Low-Glycemic-Index Diets

On the glycemic index, a Snickers bar is considered healthier than a banana. Is this a wise eating plan?

A number of books and diet doctors have recently started advocating low-glycemic-index diets. Proponents of these diets claim that foods low on the glycemic index (those that cause small increases in blood glucose levels when eaten) are healthier than foods high on this index (those that cause sharp increases in blood glucose). However, the most recent guidelines from the American Diabetes Association do not recommend the glycemic index as a useful tool for planning a healthy diet.

What the Glycemic Index Means

The glycemic index is a system for classifying carbohydrate-containing foods based on how quickly and for how long they raise blood glucose levels. Although not proven, proponents of low-glycemic-index diets believe that sharp rises in blood glucose levels are detrimental. They argue that the surge of insulin that accompanies ingestion of high-glycemic-index foods causes blood sugar to drop to below-normal levels, and this makes people feel hungry again sooner.

The glycemic index of a particular food is determined by how much it causes blood glucose to rise in the two hours after it is eaten, compared with the rise in blood glucose caused by an equivalent amount of carbohydrate in white bread. White bread has a glycemic index of 100. Foods with a glycemic index above 100, like instant rice, cause a greater increase in blood glucose than white bread; conversely, kidney beans (which have a glycemic index of 38) only raise blood glucose one third as much as white bread.

Shortcomings of the Index

Sometimes the index can encourage better food choices, but often it leads to worse ones. For example, someone on a low-glycemic-index diet might eat more fruits, vegetables, and whole grains because fiber lowers a food's glycemic index. But fat also slows carbohydrate absorption and gives some fatty foods a low value on the index, making them seem healthier than they really are. Another danger is avoiding healthy foods that are high on the glycemic index, such as corn, carrots, and raisins.

But the main problem with the index is that it often is not practical. First, glycemic index values are not listed on most food labels. Also, a food's effect on blood glucose levels depends on whether it is cooked or raw and what the person's blood glucose level is before eating it. In addition, the index considers only the amount of carbohydrates in a food, while most meals include fat and protein as well. And most important, the index rates only single foods eaten individually, but people usually eat several different foods together.

Moreover, no long-term clinical trials have examined whether a low-glycemic-index diet helps to regulate blood glucose levels or control weight, and observational studies have yielded inconsistent results.

The Bottom Line

Because people with diabetes need to control their blood glucose, the glycemic index might seem like a useful tool for helping them in their food choices. But the American Diabetes Association's nutritional guidelines state that people with diabetes do not have to restrict their food choices to those low on the glycemic index. The total amount of carbohydrate eaten each day is more important in determining the body's response to glucose than the glycemic index of each individual food eaten.

Some carbohydrates are preferred over others because they have more fiber or more vitamins and other nutrients. For instance, fruits, vegetables, legumes, whole-grain breads, and low-fat dairy products are better carbohydrate sources than candy or white bread. The most important thing is for people with diabetes to be able to recognize the size of their carbohydrate portions and to try to keep their carbohydrate intake relatively stable. In addition, some people with diabetes find that certain sources of carbohydrate, such as pizza or pasta sauce, throw their blood glucose levels off because of "hidden" sugar or fat in these foods. In the end, people with diabetes should consult a doctor or dietitian for help in designing a balanced diet.

accomplished by using less salt at the table and in cooking and by avoiding foods that are high in sodium (for example, processed meats such as sausages, cured ham, and hot dogs; canned or dried soups; ketchup; and most cheeses).

Protein. Most people with diabetes should consume about 10%

The Rewards of Lifting Weights

For people with diabetes, an exercise routine that includes some form of strength training can have surprising benefits.

Aerobic exercises such as walking or swimming are extremely beneficial for people with diabetes. These exercises can help control weight, lower blood glucose, improve cardiovascular fitness, and reduce the risk of diabetes complications. But new research shows that adding resistance exercises to your workout routine also can help protect against diabetes complications and other health problems.

A recent analysis found that resistance exercise was as effective as aerobic exercise at lowering hemoglobin A1C (HbA1c) levels. Another recent study showed that resistance exercise improved blood glucose control in older people with type 2 diabetes and had no adverse effects.

Resistance exercise has some advantages over aerobic exercise. Aerobic exercise burns calories only while you are exercising, but resistance exercise causes the body to burn more calories at rest by increasing muscle mass. In addition, resistance exercise can be done relatively quickly almost anywhere.

Age should not be a deterrent for starting a resistance exercise program. Studies have shown that older people can benefit just as much as younger ones. Resistance exercise may be even more important for older people, as it can also help reduce bone loss and prevent fractures.

What Is Resistance Exercise?

Resistance exercise is any movement that requires the body to exert or resist force. Lifting weights (either with a weight machine or with free weights such as barbells or dumbbells) is the most common type of resistance exercise. In resistance exercise, the muscles lift or move more weight than they are accustomed to, which strengthens them.

Why Is Resistance Exercise Beneficial?

Like aerobic exercise, resistance exercise lowers blood glucose; it increases the muscles' energy needs and more glucose moves from the blood into the muscles. In addition to increasing glucose utilization, resistance exercise decreases insulin resistance, body fat, blood triglyceride levels, and blood pressure.

Less research has been done on resistance exercise than on aerobic exercise in people with diabetes, but studies suggest that resistance exercise is effective. In one of these studies, published in *Diabetes Care* in 2002, 62 adults with type 2 diabetes (average age 66) were assigned to either a resistance-exercise group or a control group. People in the exercise group performed 45 minutes of supervised exercises on a weight machine three times a week for 16 weeks, while those in the control group followed their usual routine. At the end of the study, people in the exercise group lowered their HbA1c levels from 8.7% to 7.6%, and 72% were able to lower their dose of diabetes medication. By contrast, people in the control group had no change in HbA1c levels, and 42% needed to increase their dose of diabetes medications.

Is Resistance Training Safe?

Until recently, people with high blood pressure, heart disease, and arthritis

to 20% of total calories from protein. For those with nephropathy, however, reducing dietary protein to even lower levels may help slow kidney damage. High-protein, low-carbohydrate diets should be undertaken with caution, since the long-term effects of these diets on the risk of CHD and kidney dysfunction are unknown.

Alcohol. People with well-controlled diabetes can drink alcoholic beverages, as long as they do so in moderation and with food. The American Diabetes Association recommends that men drink no more than two alcoholic drinks per day, and women no more than one. (One drink is equivalent to 12 oz. of beer, 5 oz. of wine, or 1½ oz. of distilled spirits.) People with additional medical problems, such as pancreatitis (inflammation of the pancreas), advanced neuropathy, or elevated triglyceride levels, should abstain from alcohol altogether.

were advised not to lift weights because of concerns that it might worsen their condition. However, research has shown that this is not the case. Likewise, resistance training has been shown to be safe for people with diabetes, and it may be a better choice than aerobic activity for people with peripheral neuropathy or peripheral vascular disease, who cannot spend prolonged periods of time walking or jogging.

Resistance exercise with heavy weights may not be appropriate for people with proliferative diabetic retinopathy, because strenuous activity may increase damage to the eyes. However, resistance exercise with light weights is safe for nearly everyone with diabetes.

Keeping Blood Glucose Levels in Check During Exercise

People who take insulin or oral medication to control their diabetes need to protect against hypoglycemia (low blood glucose) while exercising:

- If your preworkout blood glucose level is between 100 and 250 mg/dL, it is safe for you to begin exercising. If glucose is lower than 100 mg/dL, have a carbohydrate snack such as a piece of fruit or three graham crackers before starting. If levels are higher than 250 mg/dL and you have type 1 diabetes, test your urine for ketones, and delay exercise if ketone levels are moderate or high. Do not exercise if your blood glucose levels are 300 mg/dL or higher.
- Test your blood glucose level every 30 minutes during exercise. If it starts to fall, have a snack.
- If you experience any symptoms of hypoglycemia during exercise (such as faintness, palpitations, or weakness), test your blood glucose levels immediately and, if necessary, have a snack.
- Blood glucose levels can drop hours after exercise, so test your levels immediately after your workout and again a few hours later.
- Always have a source of fast-acting carbohydrate (such as glucose tablets or hard candies) with you when exercising.

Beginning a Resistance Program

Before starting to lift weights, see your health care professional for a thorough medical examination. To get the most benefit from resistance exercise, follow these steps:

- If you have never used weights before, schedule some time with a personal trainer or fitness instructor at a gym or community center. He or she can show you how to use the equipment properly, as well as determine the appropriate weight and number of repetitions for you. In general, using light weights and doing many repetitions is the best choice.
- Because machines can help ensure good form while lifting weights, they are safer to use than dumbbells or hand weights.
- Only lift weights when someone else is nearby to offer assistance if needed.
- Before lifting, do 5 to 10 minutes of warm-up activity such as walking, jogging, or jumping jacks.
- Remember to breathe properly when lifting. Exhale when lifting the weight and inhale when releasing it. Don't hold your breath.
- Do not lift weights more frequently than every other day. Your muscles need time to recover between resistance workouts.

The calories from alcohol should be exchanged for those that would normally be allotted for fat servings. Drinks that contain smaller amounts of sugar, such as light beers and dry wines, are preferable to mixed drinks that are high in sugar.

Heavy drinking should be avoided, and those who drink should be aware that alcohol can cause weight gain (because of its high calorie content), hypoglycemia, elevated triglyceride levels, and flushing in the face, arms, and neck in some people taking oral diabetes drugs, especially chlorpropamide (Diabinese).

Exercise

Exercise is beneficial for people with diabetes: It helps lower blood glucose levels and blood pressure, improves levels of blood cholesterol and triglycerides, and provides a sense of well-being. The

American College of Sports Medicine and the American Diabetes Association recommend that people with type 2 diabetes get at least 45 minutes of aerobic exercise such as walking, cycling, or swimming three days a week, plus engage in resistance training using light weights at least twice a week. For more information on resistance training, see the feature on pages 30–31.

Exercise requires careful planning and monitoring, particularly for people who take oral medication or insulin to control their diabetes. These individuals need to check their blood glucose levels before and after exercising and may need to make adjustments to their medication or food intake to prevent blood glucose levels that are too low or too high during exercise. In addition, people with arthritis, peripheral vascular disease, or peripheral neuropathy may need to modify their exercise program to avoid foot trauma (for example, by replacing jogging with swimming or bicycling). Always be sure to talk to your doctor before beginning an exercise program or making any changes to your medication or diet.

Oral Medications

Diet and exercise may be enough to control blood glucose levels in some people with type 2 diabetes, but when the response to these measures is inadequate, oral medications are generally started. The six classes of oral drugs for diabetes are the sulfonylureas, biguanides, alpha-glucosidase inhibitors, meglitinides, thiazolidinediones, and D-phenylalanine derivatives. The chart on pages 34–35 and the text below provide an overview of these drugs.

Sulfonylureas. Sulfonylureas stimulate the pancreas to secrete more insulin. These medications are classified as first-generation or second-generation. Chlorpropamide (Diabinese) is a first-generation sulfonylurea. Second-generation drugs include glimepiride (Amaryl), glipizide (Glucotrol, Glucotrol XL), and glyburide (DiaBeta, Glynase, Micronase). The second-generation drugs are more potent than the first-generation agents and are prescribed at lower dosages.

About 85% of people with type 2 diabetes who do not achieve adequate blood glucose control with diet and exercise initially show a favorable response to a sulfonylurea. However, people with fasting blood glucose levels above 300 mg/dL rarely benefit from this class of drugs. In addition, in more than a quarter of people who initially respond to a sulfonylurea, the drug loses its effectiveness. When a sulfonylurea does not lower blood glucose levels sufficiently, metformin, an alpha-glucosidase inhibitor, or a thiazolidinedione can be added to the treatment regimen. Alternately, metformin alone may be tried as a replacement for a sulfonylurea. If all types of oral medications fail, insulin is required.

Adverse effects occur in roughly 3% of people taking a sulfonylurea. The most common and serious side effect is hypoglycemia, which is more likely to occur in debilitated elderly people, malnourished individuals, and those with pituitary, adrenal, liver, or kidney dysfunction. Alcohol, skipped meals, and exercise also can trigger hypoglycemia in people taking a sulfonylurea. If hypoglycemia occurs, the dose of the drug is usually reduced. Sulfonylureas can also cause weight gain, excessive water retention, and, occasionally, flushing after alcohol consumption.

Biguanides. Metformin (Glucophage), which is also available in an extended-release form (Glucophage XR), belongs to a class of oral medications called biguanides. These drugs act primarily by decreasing the liver's production of glucose but also increase the uptake of glucose by cells.

Metformin is used alone or in combination with a sulfonylurea, a meglitinide, an alpha-glucosidase inhibitor, a thiazolidinedione, or insulin. Some studies have shown that metformin can reduce blood glucose levels by about 20% and boost the glucose-lowering effects of a sulfonylurea by an additional 25%.

One of metformin's main advantages is that it provides another option for people with type 2 diabetes who do not achieve adequate glucose control with a sulfonylurea. In fact, metformin can be used either as a first-line oral agent (before a sulfonylurea is tried) or as a second-line agent when a sulfonylurea no longer works adequately. Additional benefits of metformin include a significant reduction in total and LDL cholesterol and triglyceride levels and no risk of hypoglycemia or weight gain. In fact, some people on metformin actually lose weight. In one study, metformin helped patients to lose an average of almost 6 lbs., most of which was body fat. Weight loss with metformin may be the result of a small decrease in appetite.

The most common side effect of metformin is diarrhea, which tends to improve with continued use of the drug. Other side effects include mild nausea, bloating, and gas. These gastrointestinal side effects occur in 30% of people. Metformin can also cause hypoglycemia when used in combination with a sulfonylurea, a meglitinide, or insulin. A buildup of lactic acid in the blood (lactic acidosis) is rare but life-threatening when it occurs. To avoid this dangerous complication, metformin should not be used in people with kidney or liver disease, heart failure, severe emphysema or

NEW RESEARCH

Moderate Drinking May Lessen Diabetes Risk

Having two to seven drinks per week may improve blood glucose levels and reduce the risk of type 2 diabetes in young and middle-aged women, two new studies show. Previous studies have shown a benefit in men and older women.

The first study analyzed the drinking habits of more than 100,000 female nurses (age 25 to 42). Ten years later, the risk of diabetes was 33% lower in women who had up to one drink per day than in teetotalers, and 58% lower in women who had one to two drinks per day. But when women had more than two drinks per day, the apparent benefits of alcohol consumption disappeared.

The second study involved 459 normal-weight and overweight female nurses (age 33 to 50). Compared with nondrinkers, women who drank moderately were more likely to have lower HbA1c and insulin levels, particularly if they were overweight. Higher insulin levels are evidence of insulin resistance, a risk factor for diabetes.

The researchers theorize that light to moderate alcohol intake may improve insulin sensitivity, but they caution that there are potential adverse effects of excessive alcohol intake.

ARCHIVES OF INTERNAL MEDICINE
Volume 163, page 1329
June 9, 2003

DIABETES CARE
Volume 26, page 1971
July 2003

Oral Blood Glucose-Lowering Medications 2004

Drug Type	Generic Name	Brand Name	Onset and Duration of Action
Sulfonylureas	chlorpropamide	Diabinese	Should be taken once a day with breakfast; peaks in 2 to 4 hours and lasts for 24 to 28 hours.
	glimepiride	Amaryl	Should be taken once a day with breakfast; peaks in 2 to 3 hours and lasts for 24 hours.
	glipizide	Glucotrol	Should be taken once or twice a day 30 minutes before a meal; peaks in 1 to 3 hours and lasts 12 to 24 hours.
	glipizide, extended release	Glucotrol XL	Should be taken once a day with breakfast; peaks in 6 to 12 hours and lasts for 24 hours.
	glyburide	DiaBeta Glynase Micronase	Should be taken once or twice a day before a meal; peaks in 4 hours and lasts for 24 hours.
Biguanides	metformin	Glucophage	Should be taken 2 to 3 times daily before meals; lasts for 12 hours.
	metformin, extended release	Glucophage XR	Should be taken with the evening meal; lasts for 24 hours.
Combination agents	glipizide and metformin glyburide and metformin rosiglitazone and metformin	Metaglip Glucovance Avandamet	Should be taken with meals; lasts for 12 hours.
Thiazolidinediones	pioglitazone rosiglitazone	Actos Avandia	These drugs should be taken once or twice a day with or without meals; they peak in 3 hours and last for 16 to 34 hours.
Meglitinide	repaglinide	Prandin	Should be taken up to 30 minutes before meals; peaks in 30 to 60 minutes and lasts for 1 to 2 hours.
D-phenylalanine derivative	nateglinide	Starlix	Should be taken 1 to 30 minutes before each meal; peaks within 1 hour and lasts a few hours.
Alpha-glucosidase inhibitors	acarbose miglitol	Precose Glyset	Should be taken just before a meal; lasts about 1 hour.

other chronic lung diseases, or high intakes of alcohol.

Alpha-glucosidase inhibitors. Acarbose (Precose) and miglitol (Glyset) inhibit alpha-glucosidase enzymes in the intestine. As a result, they delay the digestion of carbohydrates (both starches and sucrose) and blunt the peak levels of glucose and insulin in the blood after a meal. They are taken alone or in combination with a sulfonylurea, a meglitinide, metformin, a thiazolidinedione, or insulin.

Wholesale Cost* (Generic Cost)	Comments
250 mg: $96 ($64)	May be used alone or with metformin, an alpha-glucosidase inhibitor, or a thiazolidinedione. Hypoglycemia is the most worrisome side effect (particularly in the elderly, debilitated, or malnourished). May cause water retention, weight gain, constipation, diarrhea, dizziness, headache, heartburn, increased or decreased appetite, and stomach pain or discomfort. Drinking alcohol while taking chlorpropamide can cause flushing in the face, arms, and neck.
2 mg: $54 5 mg: $45 ($35) 5 mg: $43 5 mg: $84 ($78) 6 mg: $137 5 mg: $101 ($78)	May be used alone or with metformin, an alpha-glucosidase inhibitor, or a thiazolidinedione. A smaller dosage is required than with the first-generation agent, chlorpropamide. Side effects are similar to those listed for chlorpropamide above.
500 mg: $78 ($70) 500 mg: $74	May be used alone or with a sulfonylurea, a meglitinide, an alpha-glucosidase inhibitor, a thiazolidinedione, or insulin. Also helps lower total and LDL cholesterol and triglyceride levels and may help with weight control. Does not produce hypoglycemia when used alone. May cause diarrhea, nausea, bloating, and, rarely, a fatal buildup of lactic acid in the blood.
5 mg/500 mg: $94 5 mg/500 mg: $94 4 mg/500 mg: $264	See separate entries for glipizide and metformin. See separate entries for glyburide and metformin. See separate entries for rosiglitazone and metformin.
15 mg: $320 4 mg: $277	May be used alone or with a sulfonylurea, a meglitinide, metformin, an alpha-glucosidase inhibitor, or insulin. Side effects are uncommon but include fluid retention and possible heart failure. Liver tests are advised. Insulin dose may need to be decreased to avoid hypoglycemia. Full effects may require two to eight weeks of treatment.
0.5 mg: $98	May be used alone or with metformin, an alpha-glucosidase inhibitor, or a thiazolidinedione. Hypoglycemia, the most frequent side effect, is less common than with sulfonylureas.
60 mg: $105	May be used alone or with metformin. The most common side effect is hypoglycemia.
50 mg: $70 50 mg: $72	May be used alone or with a sulfonylurea, a meglitinide, metformin, a thiazolidinedione, or insulin. May cause gas, soft stools, diarrhea, and abdominal discomfort, which tend to lessen with time.

*Average wholesale prices to pharmacists for 100 tablets of the dosage listed. Costs to consumers are higher. If a generic version is available, the cost is listed in parentheses. Source: *Red Book, 2003* (Medical Economics Data, publishers).

The most common side effects—gas, diarrhea, and abdominal discomfort—tend to lessen over time, but many people are unable to tolerate these drugs because of excessive gas. When taken alone, acarbose and miglitol do not cause hypoglycemia. If hypoglycemia occurs when taking these drugs with a sulfonylurea, a meglitinide, or insulin, the condition must be treated by ingesting glucose (dextrose) or fruit juice—rather than products containing sucrose, which cannot be digested and absorbed due to the drug's inhibition of alpha-glucosidase enzymes. Acarbose and miglitol should not be used by people with inflammatory bowel disease or other serious intestinal disorders.

Meglitinides. Repaglinide (Prandin) is the only meglitinide approved by the FDA. The drug induces the pancreas to secrete insulin dependent on the amount of glucose in the blood. As a result, repaglinide has a more rapid effect on insulin levels and offers more flexibility than a sulfonylurea.

Repaglinide can be taken with metformin if either drug alone does not control blood glucose adequately. It can also be used in combination with an alpha-glucosidase inhibitor or a thiazolidinedione. Hypoglycemia, the most common side effect, occurs less often than with sulfonylureas.

Thiazolidinediones. Pioglitazone (Actos) and rosiglitazone (Avandia) are the two thiazolidinediones currently available. These drugs work by decreasing resistance of cells to the actions of insulin. Since obese people with diabetes are resistant to insulin, these individuals may benefit the most from taking a thiazolidinedione. Thiazolidinediones are used alone or in combination with a sulfonylurea, a meglitinide, metformin, an alpha-glucosidase inhibitor, or insulin.

Troglitazone (Rezulin), the first drug approved in this class, was withdrawn from the market in 2000 because of reports of rare, but severe, liver failure and related deaths. Pioglitazone and rosiglitazone are far less toxic to the liver than troglitazone. Still, the FDA recommends a blood test to measure liver function before people begin taking a thiazolidinedione and regularly thereafter.

Thiazolidinediones can cause fluid retention, which can lead to heart failure or worsen existing heart failure. The drugs can also cause rapid weight gain independent of fluid retention. In addition, the cholesterol-lowering medication cholestyramine (Questran) inhibits the absorption of thiazolidinediones and should not be taken at the same time of day. Because the full effect of a thiazolidinedione may not occur until several weeks or even months after the drug is initiated, people taking both a thiazolidinedione and insulin need to be monitored to see whether the insulin dose needs to be decreased to avoid hypoglycemia.

D-phenylalanine derivatives. Nateglinide (Starlix) is the only D-phenylalanine derivative approved by the FDA. The drug lowers blood glucose levels after meals by stimulating the rapid production of insulin by the pancreas. Nateglinide seems to be most effective when blood glucose levels after a meal are unusually high

NEW RESEARCH

More Vigorous Exercise Offers Better Heart Protection

Exercise is known to reduce the risk of heart disease and death in healthy adults, and now a study shows that physical activity such as walking helps protect the hearts of people with diabetes, too. In addition, the faster people walked, the fewer hearts attacks they had.

More than 2,800 men who developed diabetes at age 30 or older told researchers how much time they spent in leisure-time physical activity during an average week. The participants provided updated information every two years from 1986 to 1998.

Men who spent three to five hours walking briskly, two to three hours jogging, or one to two hours running each week cut their risk of cardiovascular disease by 36% and their risk of death by 43%, compared with men who did very little exercise. Also, men who walked very briskly (four miles per hour or more) for exercise were 83% less likely to have a fatal or nonfatal heart attack than men who walked at an easy pace (less than two miles per hour).

Moderate exercise offered the maximum benefit, calling into question the value of very vigorous exercise. An accompanying editorial points out that exercise is "vastly underutilized in the management of diabetes, and the majority of individuals remain sedentary or do too little exercise to achieve health benefits."

CIRCULATION
Volume 107, pages 2392 and 2435
May 20, 2003

(more than 200 mg/dL). The drug can be taken by itself or in combination with metformin.

The most common side effect is hypoglycemia. Rare side effects include upper respiratory infection, flu symptoms, dizziness, and joint pain. The drug should be used with caution in people with significant liver disease.

Insulin

More than a third of people with type 2 diabetes eventually require insulin treatment to control blood glucose levels as the severity of diabetes worsens and oral drugs lose their effectiveness. By contrast, all people with type 1 diabetes need insulin treatment to control their disease. Sulfonylureas, metformin, and thiazolidinediones may be prescribed in combination with insulin for people with type 2 diabetes.

Types of insulin. Four main types of insulin are available: rapid-acting, very rapid-acting, intermediate-acting, and long-acting. Insulin mixtures are also available.

Rapid-acting insulin (also called regular insulin) is injected 30 to 45 minutes before meals to cover the rise in blood glucose that begins about 15 minutes after food is eaten. Two very rapid-acting insulins called insulin aspart (Novolog) and insulin lispro (Humalog) are absorbed more quickly than regular insulin and begin to work within 10 to 20 minutes of injection. Unlike most other types of insulin, insulin aspart and insulin lispro are available only by prescription, since their effect on children and pregnant women is unknown.

Intermediate-acting insulins contain protamine (NPH insulin) or large, zinc-containing crystals of insulin (lente insulin); both substances slow the absorption of insulin. Long-acting insulin (ultralente insulin) has even larger zinc-insulin crystals, which further prolong the entry of insulin into the blood. Insulin glargine (Lantus), another long-acting insulin, forms crystals in fat tissue that slow its absorption. Intermediate- and long-acting insulins are usually injected once or twice a day. For an overview of the various types of insulin, see the chart on pages 38–39.

Typically, a combination of insulin types is used to treat diabetes. Regular insulin or very rapid-acting insulin is often added to intermediate- or long-acting insulin before one or more meals to reduce the after-meal increase in blood glucose. For example, in the DCCT, tight glucose control in people with type 1 diabetes was attained with injections of regular insulin before each meal, plus NPH or lente

NEW RESEARCH

Even Without Weight Loss, Exercise Improves Insulin Sensitivity

According to a recent small study, sedentary people who begin to exercise regularly, even if they don't lose weight, may still reduce their risk of insulin resistance, which increases the likelihood of type 2 diabetes and cardiovascular disease.

Eighteen adults (average age 52) without diabetes who did not exercise regularly were randomly assigned to one of three exercise groups: high intensity and low frequency (three to four days per week), high intensity and high frequency (five to seven days per week), and moderate intensity and high frequency. Exercise consisted of 30 minutes of walking at the assigned intensity and frequency. The participants were told not to alter their eating habits or try to change their body weight during the study.

After six months, participants in all three groups had improved their insulin sensitivity, even though they did not lose weight. The researchers point out that aerobic exercise is already known to reduce the risk of complications in people with type 2 diabetes; these findings suggest that exercise may also prevent type 2 diabetes in sedentary adults, including those at high risk for diabetes.

DIABETES CARE
Volume 26, page 557
March 2003

Types of Insulin 2004

Type	Drug Names	Wholesale Cost*
Rapid-acting	*Human:*	
	regular insulin (Humulin R)	10 mL vial: $28†
	regular insulin (Novolin R)	10 mL vial: $28†
	regular insulin (Novolin R Penfill)	five 1.5 mL vials: $45†
	regular insulin (Velosulin BR)	10 mL vial: $44†
Very rapid-acting	*Modified Human:*	
	insulin aspart (Novolog)	10 mL vial: $59
	insulin lispro (Humalog)	10 mL vial: $59
Intermediate-acting	*Human:*	
	lente insulin (Humulin L)	10 mL vial: $28†
	lente insulin (Novolin L)	10 mL vial: $28†
	NPH insulin (Humulin N)	10 mL vial: $28†
	NPH insulin (Novolin N)	10 mL vial: $28†
	NPH insulin (Novolin N Penfill)	five 1.5 mL vials: $45†
Long-acting	*Human:*	
	ultralente insulin (Humulin U)	10 mL vial: $28†
	Modified Human:	
	insulin glargine (Lantus)	10 mL vial: $51
Mixtures	*Human:*	
	50% NPH and 50% regular insulin (Humulin 50/50)	10 mL vial: $28†
	70% NPH and 30% regular insulin (Humulin 70/30)	10 mL vial: $28†
	70% NPH and 30% regular insulin (Novolin 70/30)	10 mL vial: $28†
	70% NPH and 30% regular insulin (Novolin 70/30 Penfill)	five 1.5 mL vials: $45†
	70% NPH and 30% regular insulin (Novolin 70/30 Innolet)	five 3 mL vials: $55†

insulin at bedtime or ultralente insulin with the evening meal.

Regular insulin or very rapid-acting insulin can be combined in the same syringe with intermediate- or long-acting insulin. A notable exception is insulin glargine, which cannot be mixed in the same syringe with other insulins. Because the longer-acting insulins can modify regular insulin, it is best to make the injection within five minutes of mixing the two insulin types.

Combining regular and NPH insulins can be simplified with the the use of premixed products. A 70/30 mixture, which contains 70% NPH and 30% regular insulin, and a 50/50 mixture, which contains 50% NPH and 50% regular insulin, are available. However, the fixed ratio of the two insulin types in these products may not be suitable for all people.

Modes of insulin administration. To be effective, insulin must be injected. It cannot be swallowed, because digestive enzymes would

Onset, Peak, and Duration	Comments
Begins to work in 30 minutes to 1 hour, peaks at 2 to 4 hours, and lasts for about 6 to 8 hours.	Injected before meals to cover the sugars absorbed from food.
Begins to work in about 10 to 20 minutes, peaks at about 2 hours, and lasts for about 4 hours.	The fastest-acting insulin on the market. Available only by prescription.
Begins working in about 1 to 4 hours, peaks at about 6 to 12 hours, and lasts for about 14 to 24 hours.	Often used in combination with rapid- or very rapid-acting insulin.
Action begins about 4 to 6 hours after injection, peaks after 18 to 28 hours, and lasts for up to 36 hours.	Best when combined with a rapid- or very rapid-acting insulin to cover the sugars absorbed from food at mealtimes.
Varies, according to type.	Convenient for people who use a mixture of NPH and regular insulin in one syringe. Helpful for those with poor dexterity or eyesight or for anyone who has problems drawing up insulin from two different bottles or reading the instructions and dosages on the bottle labels.

*Average wholesale prices to pharmacists for the vial size listed. Costs to consumers are higher. Source: *Red Book, 2003* (Medical Economics Data, publishers).

† Available without a prescription.

destroy the insulin before it reached the bloodstream. Injections are given subcutaneously (under the skin) at a site where there is fat tissue. The most common injection sites are the abdomen (except for a two-inch area around the navel), the front and outer side of the thigh, the upper part of the buttocks, and the outer side of the upper arm. A needle and syringe are most often used for insulin injection. Other methods of administering insulin include insulin pens, jet injectors, and external insulin pumps.

Insulin syringes. Injection of insulin with a needle and syringe—which, for years, was the only option—remains the predominant choice for most people receiving insulin in the United States. Fortunately, the devices currently available—disposable, lightweight syringes with shorter, ultrafine needles—have made daily injections more convenient and less painful.

One advantage of syringes is that they come in a wide variety of sizes and styles. Syringes may also be best for those who mix different types of insulin into one dose.

Insulin pens. Insulin pens combine an insulin container and syringe in one compact device. Two types are available: reusable and prefilled. With reusable pens, a cartridge of insulin is loaded into the pen, a needle is attached, the insulin dose is "dialed in," and a plunger is pressed to administer the injection. The prefilled pens are easier to use than reusable pens—they contain a built-in insulin cartridge and are discarded after the insulin is gone—but they can be more expensive.

Jet injectors. Jet injectors use a high-pressure jet of air to send a fine stream of insulin through the skin. These devices eliminate the need for needle sticks, but they are not widely used in part because they are bulky and expensive. In addition, they can be just as uncomfortable as insulin injections, causing pain and bruising.

External insulin pumps. First used in the early 1980s, the external insulin pump is a small, portable device (usually worn at the waist) that delivers insulin into the bloodstream via a small needle inserted just below the skin of the abdomen, thigh, or buttocks. The pump delivers a continuous amount of insulin throughout the day, in addition to extra doses of insulin before meals.

Studies show that people with type 1 diabetes who use the insulin pump have better blood glucose control than people who use traditional insulin injections. They also report an improvement in quality of life. People with type 2 diabetes who are having difficulty controlling their blood glucose levels may also benefit from the pump. Drawbacks of the pump include frequent blood glucose monitoring, the cost of the pump and its supplies, and an increased risk of skin infections. For more information on the external insulin pump, see the feature on pages 42–43.

Techniques under development. Researchers are working on a variety of new approaches to insulin delivery, including inhaled insulin, nasal insulin, oral insulin, and insulin patches. Inhaled insulin is considered to be the most promising.

Another approach showing promise is an implantable insulin pump, which is placed under the skin in the left side of the abdomen. Insulin is delivered in small, intermittent pulses at a constant rate through the tip of a catheter that rests within the abdominal cavity. The insulin pulses are supplemented by mealtime doses of insulin that are controlled by an external device that transmits commands to the pump.

The main advantages of implantable pumps appear to be tight

glucose control with a low risk of hypoglycemia and weight gain. Quality of life is improved, in part because needle injections are required only every few months to refill the pump. Major problems with implantable pumps include blockages at the end of the catheter, which may require replacement of the catheter, and the need to replace the pump every three years when the batteries wear out. The newest implantable pumps are designed to last seven to eight years.

Implantable insulin pumps are not yet approved by the FDA and are available only to people participating in clinical trials. To find out if any clinical trials of implantable pumps are accepting patients, visit these Web sites: www.clinicaltrials.gov, www.centerwatch.com, and www.trialscentral.org. About 1,300 people worldwide have been treated with implantable pumps.

Adverse effects of insulin. Patients taking insulin are susceptible to hypoglycemia when they administer too much insulin, delay or miss a meal, exercise without first eating a snack, or drink alcohol on an empty stomach. Consequently, insulin treatment requires careful attention to the timing of meals, exercise, and alcohol intake. Frequent tests of blood glucose at home and periodic HbA1c tests by a physician are necessary to determine the doses of insulin needed to achieve good control while limiting episodes of hypoglycemia.

Other adverse effects of insulin are loss or overgrowth of fat tissue at the injection sites, allergic reactions, and insulin resistance. Alterations in fat tissue, less common with the types of insulin used today, can be further minimized by rotating injection sites. Allergic reactions, also now rare, are managed with a desensitization procedure that involves beginning with injections of small doses of insulin and gradually increasing the dose. Insulin resistance, most often caused by the formation of antibodies against insulin, is treated by increasing the insulin dose.

Treatment of Hypoglycemia

Hypoglycemia (low blood glucose) is a potential side effect of insulin and certain oral medications, specifically the sulfonylureas, repaglinide, and nateglinide. There are two types of hypoglycemic symptoms: adrenergic and neurologic. Typical adrenergic symptoms—sweating, heart palpitations, nervousness, hunger, faintness, weakness, and numbness in the fingers and around the mouth—result when low blood glucose levels trigger the release of a hormone called epinephrine into the blood. This response helps return blood glucose levels to normal, as does the release of glucagon from the pancreas. These protective actions—particularly

NEW RESEARCH

Glucosamine/Chondroitin Safe for People With Diabetes and Arthritis

While animal studies have shown that supplements containing glucosamine can raise blood glucose levels, a new study is the first to suggest that these supplements are safe for people with both diabetes and osteoarthritis.

The study included 34 people (average age 70) with type 2 diabetes and osteoarthritis who were taking one or two diabetes medications. Twenty-two participants took a glucosamine/chondroitin combination containing 1,500 mg of glucosamine and 1,200 mg of chondroitin sulfate; the other 12 participants took a placebo.

Three months later, neither group had a significant change in hemoglobin A1c levels. One person in the supplement group discontinued treatment because of excessive flatulence.

The study did not address whether the treatment is beneficial for people with osteoarthritis, but the authors conclude that "since patients with diabetes are at risk for toxic effects from some of the current treatments for osteoarthritis (NSAIDs in particular), glucosamine may provide a safe alternative treatment for these patients."

ARCHIVES OF INTERNAL MEDICINE
Volume 163, page 1587
July 14, 2003

Are You a Good Candidate for an Insulin Pump?

Pump therapy can be a good alternative to multiple daily insulin injections for some people with diabetes.

People with type 1 diabetes, and some with type 2 diabetes, require insulin injections to control their blood glucose. Although many people get used to these insulin injections and achieve good blood glucose control, some may do better with an external insulin pump. These pumps more closely mimic the work of the pancreas. In addition, they can provide more lifestyle flexibility and require fewer needle sticks. Since insulin delivery is continuous, and since it is delivered subcutaneously (beneath the skin), the medical term for pump use is continuous subcutaneous insulin infusion.

An estimated 130,000 people in the United States currently use an external insulin pump.

How the Pump Works

An external insulin pump (illustrated on the opposite page) is a small, portable device that is usually worn on a belt or placed in a pocket, like a pager. The pump contains a small syringe, or reservoir, filled with insulin and is connected to a piece of flexible plastic tubing that leads to a small needle or a half-inch piece of plastic tubing, which is inserted just under the skin and taped in place. The needle or insert is usually placed in a fleshy part of the abdomen, thigh, or buttocks, and it must be changed every few days. The patient chooses whether to keep a little needle in place or to use the needle to insert the small end of the plastic tubing.

The pump delivers rapid-acting insulin continuously, producing a low level of insulin in the bloodstream between meals and overnight. This is called the basal rate and can be programmed to change automatically at fixed times of the day. For example, the person may need less insulin at night or more insulin during predawn hours. In addition, shortly before each meal, buttons on the pump are pressed to signal it to deliver a larger, supplemental dose (called the bolus dose) of the rapid-acting insulin. The size of the bolus dose is determined by how much the person plans to eat and what his or her blood glucose level is before the meal. Also, the bolus dose is not delivered until the person is actually eating, so the timing of meals is more flexible than when injecting long-acting insulin.

Most people find the pump comfortable to wear, even during vigorous activity. The tubing from the pump to the skin is up to 3½ feet in length and allows for a wide range of movement. The pump unit is usually waterproof or can be easily disconnected, so it can be worn while bathing or swimming. The pump and tubing can also be removed (while the needle stays in place) for brief periods, such as when dressing or exercising, or for special occasions. Traditional insulin injections are required if the pump is removed for an extended period of time.

Advantages of the Pump

The major advantages of pump therapy are ease of use, flexibility, precision, and the potential for tighter blood glucose control. The insulin dose can be adjusted without having to get out supplies and administering an injection—instead, all that is required is pushing buttons on the pump. If the basal rate is correct, people can eat on their own schedule, rather than having to eat because insulin was injected a few hours earlier and is about to take effect. Also, the pump's rate can be adjusted by as little as one tenth of a unit per hour, up or down, a level of precision that isn't possible with multiple daily injections. Additionally, the pumps have several safety features: they beep if the tubing or needle is clogged, sound an alarm when the battery runs low, and have dosage limits to prevent accidentally delivering too much insulin.

Perhaps the biggest advantage of the insulin pump is its potential for improved blood glucose control. In a recent 16-week trial of 79 people with type 1 diabetes, people using a pump had an average HbA1c level that was 0.8% lower than that of people on injected insulin therapy; though some people did much better on the pump, others' HbA1c levels improved just slightly or not at all. Pump users also reported improvements in their quality of life.

A recent analysis of 12 trials in people with type 1 diabetes showed that both average blood glucose and HbA1c levels were lower in people who used the pump than in those who used injections. Because pumps offer more precise dosing, they may also lower the amount of insulin needed. In the same study, pump users required 14% less insulin (7.6 units) per day than injection users. The researchers concluded that these differences in glucose control, although small, are significant enough to help reduce long-term complications of diabetes.

Potential Problems

Although the pump makes insulin delivery easier, it certainly doesn't do the entire job. Blood glucose levels must be checked frequently throughout the day to determine the size of the bolus doses and to make sure the pump is actually delivering the insulin properly. Since the pump uses only rapid-acting insulin, any sort of malfunction—for example, a detached needle—causes a rapid drop in blood insulin levels, and extremely high blood glucose levels can develop within hours. The built-in alarms are helpful but not foolproof.

Early studies found that people using pumps were more likely than injection users to have episodes of hypoglycemia; however, more recent research suggests that pump users may have fewer episodes (60% fewer, in one study). The same is true for diabetic ketoacidosis: While early studies suggested that it was more frequent in pump users, more recent studies show it occurs with equal frequency in pump users and injection users. Possible explanations are that doctors are getting better at teaching people how to use pumps properly and at determining who is and who is not a good candidate for pump treatment.

Skin infections are more common with pumps than with injections. Because the tubing and needle stay in place for several days, bacteria have a chance to grow at the site of the needle insertion. These infections are usually mild and go away on their own once the insertion site is changed. Occasionally, you may need to take an oral antibiotic or have a doctor drain the infected area.

Expense is another potential disadvantage of the pump. The initial cost is between $5,000 and $6,000 for the unit itself, and monthly expenses for supplies are about $482 (compared with $335 for injections). Most insurance companies cover the cost of the pump and supplies, but you will need a prescription from your doctor.

Finally, although most people are extremely happy with the freedom their pump provides, some do not like having a device attached to them. Others may notice the pump and ask what it is, so pump users need to be comfortable with people knowing that they have diabetes.

Who Is a Good Candidate?

The first reason *not* to use a pump is not wanting to. Some of the least successful pump users are those who tried it because someone else insisted—such as a spouse or doctor. Pump therapy is not recommended for people who do not practice good self-care. Significant psychological problems, such as psychosis, severe depression, or alcoholism, can prevent a person from keeping up with the demands of pump therapy. Finally, people should not use the pump if they are overly worried about using the device during contact sports or sexual activities (even after receiving training in the use of the pump and counseling).

The best candidates for pump therapy are people with a positive and realistic attitude toward the pump who require three or four daily insulin injections, have established good self-care patterns, and perhaps have an unpredictable daily schedule. Specifically, pump therapy is most likely to be successful in people who are willing to:
• test their blood glucose at least three to four times per day (including, perhaps, during the night);
• carry supplies (pump batteries, insulin cartridges, backup insulin, and syringes) with them at all times;
• make sure the pump is working correctly and know how to operate it;
• analyze blood glucose readings and adjust insulin doses as needed;
• determine the size of the bolus dose based on the amount of carbohydrates in a meal;
• work with a health care team to make any necessary adjustments; and
• check ketones when blood glucose levels are high.

If you are interested in trying pump therapy, discuss the option with your doctor. Keep in mind that the pump requires an added level of commitment and responsibility.

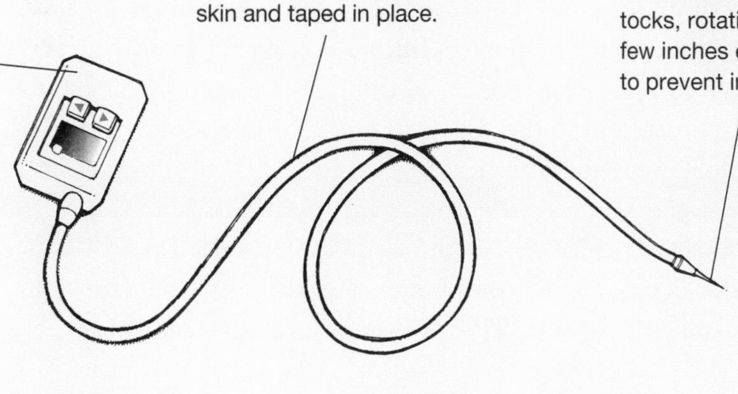

Housed in a lightweight **plastic case** (about the size of a pager) are the battery-operated pump itself, a small syringe or reservoir for the insulin, and a computer chip that allows the user to program how much insulin is delivered.

Insulin is sent through a thin, flexible, **plastic tube** to a fine needle inserted beneath the skin and taped in place.

Most people place the **needle** (or piece of plastic tubing) beneath the skin of the abdomen, thigh, or buttocks, rotating the site a few inches every three days to prevent infection.

the release of glucagon—are often lost after having diabetes for 5 to 10 years.

Though unpleasant, adrenergic symptoms alert people with diabetes that they need to eat some sugar-containing food or liquid to raise their blood glucose levels rapidly. However, these symptoms of hypoglycemia may be diminished or absent in people who are taking beta-blockers or have diabetes-related nerve damage.

Neurologic symptoms—headache, lack of coordination, double vision, inappropriate behavior, and confusion—are a greater danger because people may become confused before they can treat themselves (and thus need another person's assistance). Extreme hypoglycemia can cause seizures, coma, and, in rare cases, permanent brain damage and death.

Hypoglycemia is treated with 10 to 15 g of fast-acting carbohydrates—foods or liquids that contain sugars that are rapidly absorbed into the bloodstream. Some examples are 4 oz. of orange juice, 6 oz. of nondiet soda, five to seven hard candies, or two to five glucose tablets. People with diabetes should always have one of these fast-acting carbohydrates on hand. Avoid using foods like chocolate or nuts to treat hypoglycemia; they contain carbohydrates but take longer to digest because they also contain fat.

Glucagon injections can also rapidly raise blood glucose levels. Some people with diabetes keep glucagon in the refrigerator. Friends and family can be trained to inject glucagon, in case the person with diabetes experiences a severe episode of hypoglycemia and is not alert enough to eat anything.

Pancreas and Islet Transplants

A pancreas transplant is considered only for people with type 1 diabetes when the condition is so severe that it becomes debilitating or even life-threatening. The procedure was first developed in 1967 at the University of Minnesota, but few transplants were performed until the late 1970s. The procedure involves implanting a pancreas from a deceased donor into the pelvic region of the person with diabetes. Pancreatic veins are attached to the iliac vein (which returns blood to the heart from the lower abdomen), allowing insulin produced by the transplanted organ to enter the circulatory system. About 540 pancreas transplants are performed in the United States each year.

The one-year success rate for pancreas transplants is 78%; the one-year patient survival rate is 97%. When successful, pancreas transplants return blood glucose levels to normal and free patients from daily insulin injections and rigid dietary control; however, the procedure has several drawbacks. Transplant patients must trade daily insulin injections for daily doses of immunosuppressive drugs, which help prevent the body from rejecting the new organ. These drugs must be taken for life and have a wide range of serious side effects, including a greater risk of infections and cancer, elevated blood pressure and blood cholesterol, and more rapid deterioration of kidney function. In addition, a pancreas transplant does not appear to halt or reverse established diabetes complications, such as nephropathy, retinopathy, or macrovascular disease.

A combined pancreas/kidney transplant is considered when people with severe type 1 diabetes also have end-stage kidney disease. About 870 combined pancreas/kidney transplants are performed in the United States each year. This procedure eliminates the need for both dialysis and daily insulin injections. A combined pancreas/kidney transplant is more likely to be successful than a pancreas transplant alone. The one-year success rate for a combined transplant is 83%; the one-year patient survival rate is 95%. Another option for people with kidney failure is to have a kidney transplant only, preferably from a living donor (people can live with only one of their two kidneys). The one-year patient survival rate for this procedure is 95%.

One drawback to a combined pancreas/kidney transplant is the need for higher doses of immunosuppressive drugs than for a pancreas transplant alone. And, as with a solo pancreas transplant, there is no evidence that a combined pancreas/kidney transplant improves any existing diabetes complications.

The ideal treatment for type 1 diabetes may be transplantation of pancreatic islets that contain insulin-secreting beta cells. In this procedure, pancreata from deceased donors are treated with an enzyme that breaks up connective tissue. The islets are then separated from the remaining pancreatic tissue and transplanted into the patient's kidney, abdominal cavity, or liver. This approach has been hampered by difficulties in obtaining the large number of donor islets needed to secrete enough insulin and by the rapid decline in function of the transplanted islets, possibly due to damage by the immunosuppressive drugs used to prevent rejection.

A possible way to overcome these problems may be to produce insulin-secreting cells from stem cells. Another approach was developed by a group of Canadian researchers. They transplanted large numbers of pancreatic islets into the livers of seven people with type 1 diabetes. To prevent rejection, they used a combination of immunosuppressive drugs that do not contain corticosteroids. One year

NEW RESEARCH

Diabetic Retinopathy Treatment Preserves Vision Long-Term

Laser photocoagulation appears to help people with diabetic retinopathy maintain good vision for up to 20 years, according to a follow-up to the Early Treatment Diabetic Retinopathy Study.

In the original study, which ended in 1989, more than 3,700 people with early diabetic retinopathy were assigned to laser photocoagulation in one eye and no treatment in the other eye. Five years later, only 4% of eyes (and 1% of patients with proliferative retinopathy) had severe vision loss.

For this study, which is the first to provide data on the long-term effects of early photocoagulation, researchers at Johns Hopkins examined the eyes of 71 people from the original group.

Thirteen to 20 years after treatment, no surviving participant had severe vision loss, and 20% had moderate vision loss. Forty-two percent had 20/20 vision or better, and 84% had 20/40 vision or better. All of the participants eventually developed proliferative retinopathy and required photocoagulation in the untreated eye, and most required repeat photocoagulation in the study eye.

These findings emphasize both the importance of early treatment of diabetic retinopathy and the need for ongoing eye exams.

OPHTHALMOLOGY
Volume 110, page 1683
September 2003

after the transplant, all seven patients were able to control their blood glucose levels without the need for insulin injections. Studies of this technique are being conducted at a number of medical centers. Although promising, this approach is still experimental.

Alternative Treatments

Alternative therapies to manage diabetes have grown in popularity, but there is little or no evidence that any of them are as effective as oral diabetes drugs or insulin in controlling blood glucose or preventing diabetes complications. Alternative therapies being marketed for blood glucose control include chromium, *Gymnema sylvestre,* and vanadium. Alpha-lipoic acid, evening primrose oil, ginkgo biloba, and chelation therapy are purported to treat or prevent the major complications of diabetes.

Individuals wishing to try alternative therapies should consult with their physician beforehand. In addition, the therapies should be used in addition to—not instead of—the prescribed treatment regimen.

TREATMENT OF DIABETES COMPLICATIONS

If diabetes complications develop, they must be treated along with the diabetes itself.

Retinopathy

When people with diabetic retinopathy develop proliferative retinopathy or macular edema, a procedure called laser photocoagulation can help halt or retard vision loss. Because laser photocoagulation is effective only at certain stages in the progression of diabetic retinopathy, annual dilated eye exams by an ophthalmologist are important to identify adverse changes in the eyes.

Proliferative retinopathy is treated with a particular type of laser photocoagulation called panretinal photocoagulation, which uses a laser to make hundreds of tiny scars over the retina. Macular edema is treated with focal laser photocoagulation, in which the laser is directed at only one area of the retina. For more information on these two procedures, see the feature on the opposite page.

If the extent or location of the retinopathy makes photocoagulation ineffective, or if the vitreous humor of the eye is too clouded with blood, vision may be improved with vitrectomy, a surgical procedure that removes the vitreous humor and replaces it with a saline solution. Roughly 70% of people who undergo vitrectomy notice

A Technique To Combat Worsening Eyesight

The risk of vision loss from diabetic retinopathy can be dramatically reduced with laser photocoagulation.

The best way to avoid diabetic retinopathy is to manage your diabetes effectively. Steps to take include controlling your blood glucose, blood pressure, and blood cholesterol and quitting smoking if you smoke. However, if diabetic retinopathy develops and macular edema or proliferative retinopathy occurs (both of which can impair vision), your risk of vision loss can be minimized with an outpatient procedure called laser photocoagulation. Because photocoagulation is effective only if macular edema or proliferative retinopathy is detected at certain stages, it is important to get an annual dilated eye exam, even if you are free from symptoms.

Focal Laser Photocoagulation

Macular edema occurs when blood vessels in the retina leak and extra fluid accumulates in the macula, causing blurred vision. For people with this condition, focal laser photocoagulation may dry up the fluid by treating the leaky blood vessels.

Before the procedure, the patient receives anesthetic drops on the surface of the eye to be treated. The doctor then aims a laser directly at the leaking blood vessels that are causing the edema. Some people see shimmering lights or flashes shortly after the procedure, and vision may be somewhat blurry for a day to several weeks afterward. It may take weeks or months for the swelling in the macula to dissipate and for vision to return to preprocedure levels. Many people require up to four sessions of photocoagulation, two to four months apart.

Panretinal Photocoagulation

Proliferative retinopathy is characterized by the growth of small, fragile new blood vessels in the eye. If one of these blood vessels bursts, the result is severe bleeding (vitreous hemorrhage) that can block vision. To slow the effects of proliferative retinopathy, physicians use a procedure called panretinal photocoagulation.

With this procedure, the physician places an anesthetic drop on the eye and uses a laser to make hundreds of spots over the entire retina (except for the macula), rather than directing the laser at only one area of the retina. The laser helps to shrink and eliminate existing new blood vessels, may prevent new blood vessel formation, and reduces the chance of further bleeding by about 50%. A common side effect is mild eye discomfort, which usually can be relieved with acetaminophen (Tylenol), aspirin, or ibuprofen (Advil, Motrin). Vision may worsen immediately after the procedure but usually improves to pretreatment levels over the next few weeks or months. Typically, patients require multiple treatment sessions.

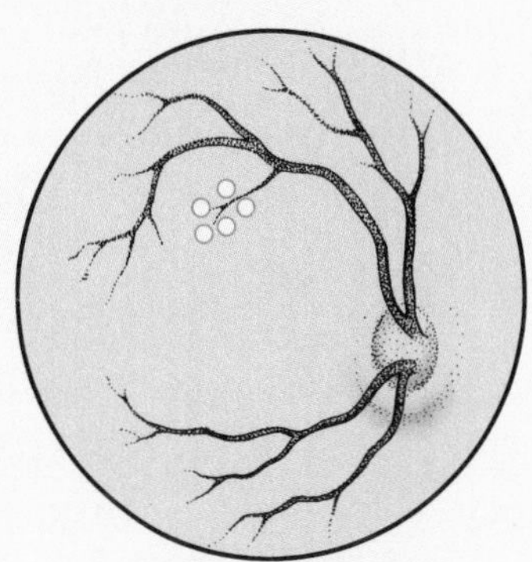

Focal laser photocoagulation

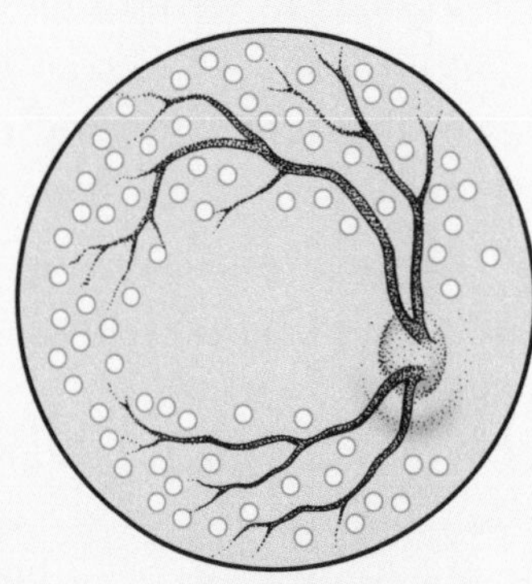

Panretinal photocoagulation

an improvement or stabilization of their eyesight, and some recover enough vision to resume reading as well as driving.

Nephropathy

Four strategies are used to prevent and slow the progression of nephropathy. The first three are tight glucose control, treating high blood pressure, and restricting protein in the diet. The fourth and most recent strategy is treatment with an ACE inhibitor, a type of drug commonly prescribed to treat high blood pressure.

ACE inhibitors slow the progression of kidney disease to kidney failure independent of their effects on blood pressure. These drugs work by slowing the production of a hormone called angiotensin. This hormone elevates the pressure across the walls of the small blood vessels in the glomeruli, where blood is filtered in the kidneys. Researchers believe that even in the absence of high blood pressure, abnormally high pressure in the glomeruli of people with diabetes can gradually destroy blood vessels in the kidney.

Two ACE inhibitors, captopril (Capoten) and enalapril (Vasotec), have been shown to slow kidney damage in the early stages of the disease. This finding has led researchers to recommend treatment with an ACE inhibitor in people with diabetes who have microalbuminuria, the first sign of kidney disease. Other researchers believe that ACE inhibitors will delay the onset of kidney disease if prescribed as soon as diabetes is diagnosed, but further studies are needed to determine the value of this approach.

A nonproductive cough is a common side effect of ACE inhibitors and may be intolerable for some people. These individuals can be treated instead with an angiotensin II receptor blocker, such as irbesartan (Avapro), losartan (Cozaar), or valsartan (Diovan). Angiotensin II receptor blockers prevent the actions of angiotensin by inhibiting its binding to receptors.

Anemia, which leads to weakness and fatigue, almost always occurs in people with chronic kidney failure. It can be improved with the use of erythropoietin, a hormone that stimulates the production of red blood cells.

Many medications are excreted from the body via the kidneys. In kidney failure, the doses of such drugs must be decreased to avoid their buildup to toxic levels. Kidney dialysis is usually initiated when kidney function deteriorates to less than 10% of normal—a condition called end-stage kidney disease.

Neuropathy

Improved control of blood glucose levels is the first step in the treatment of neuropathy, but it is often difficult to treat the symptoms associated with this condition.

Amitriptyline (Elavil, Endep), usually used to treat depression, is the most effective medication for relieving the symptoms of peripheral neuropathy. It works by making more norepinephrine available to nerve cells. (Norepinephrine is a neurotransmitter, a chemical that carries messages between nerve cells.)

NEW RESEARCH

More Aggressive Blood Pressure Control Needed in Diabetes

Even though good blood pressure control can help people with diabetes avoid long-term complications, high blood pressure may not be treated aggressively enough in this group of people, according to a recent study.

Researchers analyzed the medical records of 800 male veterans with high blood pressure; 34% also had diabetes. Blood pressures of 140/90 mm Hg or higher were found among 66% of the men without diabetes and 73% of the men with diabetes. Few participants with diabetes had blood pressures of 130/85 mm Hg or lower; the current recommended level for people with diabetes is below 130/80 mm Hg.

The study also showed that at each doctor visit from 1990 to 1995, people with diabetes were less likely than those without diabetes to be prescribed a new blood pressure-lowering medication or to have a change in their existing treatment.

The authors point out that the data were collected before the current recommendations for tight control of blood pressure in people with diabetes were introduced. However, they feel that the findings are still noteworthy because other studies "have suggested that there have not been any major changes in physicians' hypertension practices over the past 10 years."

DIABETES CARE
Volume 26, page 355
February 2003

In some individuals, amitriptyline produces troublesome side effects—drowsiness, urinary retention (the inability to empty the bladder completely), and a severe drop in blood pressure upon standing. These effects can be minimized by taking the drug at bedtime, as well as by starting with a small dose that is gradually increased. One study found that desipramine (Norpramin), another antidepressant, may be almost as effective as amitriptyline in relieving the symptoms of peripheral neuropathy and has fewer adverse effects.

Gabapentin (Neurontin) is another option, either used alone or in combination with amitriptyline. Gabapentin is an anticonvulsant approved for epilepsy; it is generally well tolerated. When side effects occur (typically drowsiness and confusion), they usually can be minimized by adjusting the dosage. According to recently published studies, gabapentin should be used for peripheral neuropathy when antidepressant drugs are ineffective or produce significant side effects.

Autonomic neuropathy can damage nerves that supply the gastrointestinal tract, resulting in symptoms such as nausea, vomiting, and diarrhea. Eating frequent, small, low-fat meals instead of three large meals a day can help prevent nausea and vomiting, which is caused by poor emptying of the stomach. Stomach emptying can also be facilitated by the drug metoclopramide (Reglan, Octamide PFS) or the antibiotic erythromycin. Diarrhea sometimes responds to antibiotics such as tetracycline (which counteract the overgrowth of intestinal bacteria that may contribute to diarrhea) or conventional antidiarrheal drugs.

Autonomic neuropathy often leads to erectile dysfunction in men. (Erectile dysfunction can also be due to other health conditions, such as vascular disease or prostate disorders, or it can have a psychological cause.) If nerves in the penis are damaged by diabetes or some other health condition, the penis may not be able to retain the blood required to create and maintain an erection. Fortunately, urologists can help men with this problem achieve an erection. These doctors can prescribe vasoactive drugs that are injected into the penis, alprostadil capsules that are inserted into the urethra, or devices that temporarily create a vacuum around the penis. In addition, oral erectile dysfunction drugs, such as sildenafil (Viagra) and vardenafil (Levitra), or surgical implants may help men with diabetes-related erectile dysfunction. Testosterone therapy may be an option for men whose testes do not produce enough testosterone. But if neuropathy or vascular disease is

NEW RESEARCH

Early Kidney Damage May Regress in Some People

Microalbuminuria, the presence of small amounts of the protein albumin in the urine, is often thought to be a sign of inevitable kidney problems in people with type 1 diabetes. However, microalbuminuria may be more likely to resolve than to worsen, according to a recent study. Even more encouraging, certain modifiable factors appear to be associated with the regression of microalbuminuria.

Researchers followed 386 people (age 15 to 44) with type 1 diabetes and microalbuminuria for six years. At the end of the study, 58% of the participants had normal levels of albumin in their urine, while only 19% had progressed to more severe proteinuria, the next step in the development of kidney disease.

Regression of microalbuminuria was most likely to occur in participants who had HbA1c levels of less than 8%, systolic blood pressures of less than 115 mm Hg, and healthy levels of cholesterol and triglycerides.

An accompanying editorial states that this study provides "welcome documentation that a widely accepted surrogate marker for the progression of [kidney] disease can be favorably influenced." Research is needed to determine whether the same is true for people with type 2 diabetes.

THE NEW ENGLAND JOURNAL OF MEDICINE
Volume 348, pages 2285 and 2349
June 5, 2003

The Benefits of Combating Depression

Depression is common in people with diabetes. Fortunately, treating depression can improve not only mood but also blood glucose control.

Depression and diabetes is an all-too-common, and potentially serious, combination. Many studies have found that depression appears twice as often in people with diabetes as in the general population. Recently, an analysis of 42 studies showed that 11% of people with diabetes had major depression and 31% had at least some symptoms of depression.

Depression can interfere with the ability to manage diabetes by making people less likely to follow dietary recommendations, take medications properly, or test their blood glucose levels regularly. People with both conditions also are more likely to have elevated hemoglobin A1c (HbA1c) levels and diabetes complications. So if depression is present, its treatment is an important component of managing diabetes and its complications.

The Diabetes-Depression Link

Diabetes and depression are clearly related, but which comes first—the diabetes or the depression? There are three major theories, and more than one may play a role in any given person.

One theory proposes that hormonal effects of diabetes or its treatment induce depression. These effects may include increased production of cortisol or changes in levels of neurotransmitters such as serotonin and norepinephrine.

A second theory says that the hardships of dealing with a chronic condition like diabetes can cause depression. Evidence for this comes from an association between depression and many chronic medical conditions besides diabetes. Also, people who are aware they have diabetes are four times more likely to be depressed than people who are unaware they have the condition.

A third theory is that the depression plays some part in causing type 2 diabetes. In most people with both type 2 diabetes and depression, depressive symptoms begin long before diabetes is diagnosed. In these people, insulin resistance (the reduced ability of the body to respond to insulin) that results from major depression may eventually induce diabetes in susceptible individuals. Also, depression may lead to low physical activity levels and poor dietary habits that can contribute to diabetes.

How Improved Mood Helps Control Diabetes

Depression can have a negative impact on the ability to manage diabetes, but fortunately, treatment of depression can improve not only depressive symptoms but also blood glucose control. One study found that people with type 2 diabetes who underwent 10 weeks of psychotherapy had lower HbA1c levels than people in a control group after six months (9.5% vs. 10.9%). In another study, treatment with the antidepressant fluoxetine (Prozac) was associated with a 0.4% decrease in HbA1c levels after eight weeks of treatment; while this reduction was not statistically significant, researchers speculate that, because HbA1c measures average blood glucose levels over a two- to three-month period, longer treatment with fluoxetine would result in greater improvements in blood glucose control.

Depression treatment may improve diabetes control in a number of ways. First, improved mood may lead to better eating and sleep habits and increased physical activity—all important factors for diabetes management. Also, improvements in mood may result in biochemical changes (such as decreased cortisol levels, improved neurotransmitter function, or greater responsiveness to insulin) that can help with blood glucose control.

Treatments for Depression

The two main treatments for depression are psychotherapy and antidepressant medication, and a combination of both is more effective than either treatment alone. Moderate

the cause of erectile dysfunction, treatment with testosterone will be ineffective.

Diabetic Foot Problems

One fifth of all hospitalizations for diabetes are for foot infections, and 86,000 amputations are performed each year because of diabetes complications. Proper foot care can eliminate or greatly reduce these risks.

exercise also can improve symptoms of depression.

Psychotherapy. This treatment is an effective option for people with mild to moderate depression. It involves talking to a mental health professional (a psychiatrist, psychologist, psychotherapist, psychiatric social worker, or psychiatric nurse specialist) in order to identify factors, such as destructive patterns of thinking or acting, that contribute to depression. The therapist may also help the patient to learn coping skills, new patterns of behavior, stress management, and relaxation techniques. Such measures can help relieve current depression and prevent bouts in the future. A drawback, however, is that psychotherapy can take six to eight weeks (or even longer) to produce a noticeable improvement in symptoms.

To find a mental health professional who practices psychotherapy, ask your doctor for a referral or contact the American Psychological Association at 800-964-2000. This organization can put you in touch with your state's psychological association, which can then refer you to a psychologist in your area. You may also be able to obtain contact information for psychotherapists from a nearby hospital or your health insurance company.

Antidepressant medication. For mild to severe forms of depression, medication is effective about 70% of the time. Medication tends to produce benefits more quickly (usually within four to six weeks) and is easier to administer than psychotherapy. Researchers believe that antidepressants work by altering levels of neurotransmitters in the brain, particularly serotonin. However, in some people, these drugs can also cause adverse effects, like weight gain and rapid heart rate. The selective serotonin reuptake inhibitors (SSRIs), which include fluoxetine, paroxetine (Paxil), and sertraline (Zoloft), may be the best option for people with diabetes.

Your primary care physician or a psychiatrist can prescribe antidepressants and determine which one may be appropriate for you. If you are interested in seeing a psychiatrist, ask for a referral from your primary care physician or go to the American Medical Association's Web site (www.ama-assn.org), where you can search for a doctor who specializes in psychiatry. Local hospitals and your health insurance company also have listings of psychiatrists in your area.

Exercise. You also might want to talk with your doctor about an exercise program. In addition to improving blood glucose control, many studies have demonstrated that exercise can improve mood. One recent report even showed that an aerobic exercise program is as effective as an antidepressant medication in the treatment of major depression in older people.

Moderate exercise appears to improve depression by decreasing stress and tension while enhancing energy. The appropriate amount and type of exercise depend on a number of factors, including your fitness level and overall health, so consult your doctor before initiating an exercise program. However, almost any form of exercise will do, including brisk walking, jogging, weight lifting, riding a bicycle, swimming, playing golf, or even gardening.

How To Recognize Depression

According to the American Psychiatric Association's *Diagnostic and Statistic Manual of Mental Disorders IV*, a person is suffering from major depression if he or she exhibits either the first or second of the following nine symptoms, in addition to at least four others, continuously for two weeks or more:

- Depressed mood;
- A loss of pleasure and interest in activities previously enjoyed;
- Significant changes in appetite and weight (a gain or loss of weight unrelated to dieting);
- Insomnia, early-morning waking, or oversleeping;
- Fatigue or decreased energy;
- Physical symptoms of restlessness or being slowed down;
- Feelings of excessive guilt or worthlessness;
- Difficulty thinking or concentrating, or indecisiveness; and
- Thoughts of suicide or death, or suicide attempts.

Everyone with diabetes, but especially those with neuropathy or poor circulation, should make a routine of good foot care. This routine involves inspecting each foot daily and carefully treating and monitoring even the most trivial cut or abrasion. When they occur, abrasions should be washed with warm water and soap, cleaned with a mild antiseptic (for example, Bactine), and covered with a dry, sterile dressing and paper tape. Ulcers are extremely serious and must be brought to the attention of a doctor immediately.

Toenails should be neatly trimmed, cut straight across rather than rounded at the ends. And at least twice a year, each foot should be examined by a physician or podiatrist.

Macrovascular Disease

With few exceptions, the management of macrovascular disease is the same for people with diabetes as for the general population. High levels of blood cholesterol and high blood pressure—major risk factors for macrovascular disease—are initially treated with diet and other lifestyle measures in an effort to bring these conditions under control without medication. In fact, many of these lifestyle measures—for example, a low-fat, high-carbohydrate diet, weight loss, and exercise—are the same as the ones recommended by the American Diabetes Association for people with diabetes. Medication is needed when elevated blood cholesterol or blood pressure persists despite strict adherence to lifestyle measures. Targets are less than 100 mg/dL for LDL cholesterol and less than 130/80 mm Hg for blood pressure.

To lower total and LDL cholesterol levels in people with diabetes, statins or bile acid sequestrants are often prescribed. The statins include atorvastatin (Lipitor), fluvastatin (Lescol), lovastatin (Mevacor), pravastatin (Pravachol), simvastatin (Zocor), and the newly approved rosuvastatin (Crestor). The bile acid sequestrants are cholestyramine (Questran), colesevelam (Welchol), and colestipol (Colestid). A recently approved drug called ezetimibe (Zetia) can also help lower total and LDL cholesterol levels, when used alone or in combination with a statin.

Statins are the medication of choice because they are more effective and easier to take than bile acid sequestrants. Two large studies have shown a significant reduction in cardiovascular events (for example, heart attacks and strokes) when people with diabetes and known CHD lowered their cholesterol levels with a statin. Nicotinic acid (niacin), the most effective medication to raise HDL cholesterol levels, is recommended less often for people with diabetes because it can elevate blood glucose levels.

Triglyceride levels above 200 mg/dL are most effectively treated with fenofibrate (Lofibra, Tricor) or gemfibrozil (Lopid). More modest elevations in triglycerides may be treated with one of the statins, which do not lower triglyceride levels as much as gemfibrozil or fenofibrate but are far more effective in reducing total and LDL cholesterol levels.

The most commonly used blood pressure-lowering medications

NEW RESEARCH

Heart Disease May Appear Earlier in People with Diabetes

Doctors have long known that diabetes increases a person's risk of coronary heart disease (CHD). Now, a study has shown—using a relatively new and sensitive technique—that CHD can be detected at a young age in people with diabetes.

Researchers used electron-beam computed tomography (EBCT) to examine the coronary arteries of more than 30,000 adults (age 30 to 90) with no symptoms of heart disease. EBCT can detect calcium deposits found in some types of plaques that build up along the inner walls of the coronary arteries. Higher calcium scores mean more plaques and a higher risk of heart attack.

Men and women with diabetes had higher calcium scores than people without diabetes in most age groups, including those younger than age 40. Other studies have shown that high calcium scores are so common among older people that these findings are not useful in predicting their risk of CHD.

The researchers suggest that EBCT might be valuable in determining the risk of CHD in young people with diabetes.

JOURNAL OF THE AMERICAN COLLEGE OF CARDIOLOGY
Volume 41, page 578
March 19, 2003

are diuretics, beta-blockers, ACE inhibitors, and calcium channel blockers. Which drug is prescribed depends on many factors, including possible side effects and cost.

An ACE inhibitor is usually the preferred drug in people with diabetes because it can both lower blood pressure and help protect the kidneys from nephropathy. The Heart Outcomes Prevention Evaluation (HOPE) study showed that treatment with the ACE inhibitor ramipril (Altace) significantly reduced the number of cardiovascular complications over a five-year period in people with diabetes and one other risk factor for CHD.

Diuretics and beta-blockers are also sometimes used to treat high blood pressure in people with diabetes. However, these drugs need to be used with caution—diuretics can raise blood glucose levels and beta-blockers can block the warning symptoms of hypoglycemia. Beta-blockers work by impeding the action of epinephrine, the hormone responsible for producing symptoms such as sweating, nervousness, and hunger that forewarn people of hypoglycemia. In the absence of these symptoms, blood glucose could fall to dangerously low levels without the person being aware of it.

Diabetes produces changes in the blood that make it more prone to clotting, thereby increasing the risk of heart attacks and strokes. Aspirin, which reduces the tendency of the blood to clot, has been shown to lower the incidence of heart attacks in people with or without known heart disease. In fact, an Israeli study found that taking aspirin decreased the risk of death from heart disease and other causes in people with diabetes and CHD even more than it did in people who had CHD but no diabetes. Effective dosages range from 80 to 325 mg (one baby aspirin or one adult aspirin daily).

Angina—chest pain due to reduced blood flow to the heart—can be treated with medication or surgery. Most often angina is the result of the buildup of plaques in the coronary arteries. Nitrate drugs (such as nitroglycerin) can alleviate angina when it occurs. Nitrates can also be used preventively when engaging in activities that are likely to cause chest pain, such as walking or playing tennis. Long-acting nitrates often help to prevent angina over the long term.

Bypass surgery and angioplasty are surgical treatments for angina. In bypass surgery, the left internal mammary artery (which usually supplies blood to the chest wall) is redirected to a site beyond the narrowed portion of a coronary artery. Alternatively, a portion of a vein from the leg is surgically attached on both sides of the blockage. In either case, blood flow is rerouted through the new vessel, which passes around the narrowed segment of artery.

NEW RESEARCH

Intensive Risk Factor Intervention Reduces Heart Attack Risk

People with type 2 diabetes are less likely to have a heart attack or stroke if they receive intensive therapy to lower risk factors for cardiovascular disease, a new study shows.

Researchers randomly assigned 80 patients (average age 56) with type 2 diabetes and microalbuminuria to standard therapy and another 80 patients to intensive therapy aimed at tight control of blood glucose levels, cholesterol levels, and blood pressure. Participants receiving intensive therapy were encouraged to eat a diet containing less than 30% of calories from fat and to exercise at least 30 minutes three to five times a week. High blood pressure, elevated lipids, and insufficiently controlled blood glucose levels were treated with medications. The participants also took a multivitamin and 150 mg of aspirin per day.

After nearly eight years, participants in the standard-therapy group were twice as likely to develop cardiovascular disease as people in the intensive-therapy group. The intensive therapy group also developed less kidney disease, retinopathy, and autonomic neuropathy.

The study authors acknowledge that multiple-risk-factor intervention is difficult, but they point out that the benefits of such intensive therapy are great.

THE NEW ENGLAND JOURNAL OF MEDICINE
Volume 348, page 383
January 30, 2003

In angioplasty, a catheter with a balloon at its tip is inserted into the femoral artery in the groin and guided to the coronary arteries in the heart. Once the catheter is positioned inside the narrowed portion of the artery, the cardiologist inflates the balloon several times to squeeze the plaque against the wall of the artery, thus widening the arterial opening and increasing blood flow to the heart. (In most angioplasty procedures, a metal tube, called a stent, is implanted in the artery to keep it propped open.)

The choice between bypass surgery and angioplasty depends on many factors, including the extent of CHD and the location of the blockage. Studies have shown an advantage for bypass surgery in people with diabetes who can withstand this more invasive procedure (bypass surgery also requires a longer recovery period than angioplasty). One ongoing study of more than 1,800 patients found that for people with diabetes, survival at seven years was significantly better with bypass surgery (76%) than with angioplasty (56%).

Immediately after a heart attack, people with diabetes may be able to lower their risk of death by regularly taking insulin. In a recent study of heart attack survivors (most had type 2 diabetes), normal blood glucose levels were maintained in one group of patients with infusions of insulin and glucose in the hospital. These individuals then gave themselves insulin injections four times a day for at least three months. Another group received conventional care for their diabetes. After a year, the overall death rate in the intensive-treatment group was 19%, compared with 26% in the conventional-treatment group—a 29% reduction.

A review of studies found that people with diabetes also benefit from beta-blockers and ACE inhibitors after a heart attack. Beta-blockers given promptly after a heart attack reduced the risk of death by 37% in patients with diabetes vs. 13% in people without diabetes; long-term treatment reduced the risk of dying by 48% in diabetic patients vs. 33% in nondiabetics. ACE inhibitors, especially when given within 24 to 36 hours of a heart attack, had similar results. One study found that taking ACE inhibitors within 36 hours of a heart attack reduced the risk of death by up to 44% in patients with type 1 diabetes and 25% in those with type 2 diabetes. ■

GLOSSARY

ACE inhibitors—Commonly prescribed to treat high blood pressure, this class of drugs also slows the progression of kidney disease in people with diabetes.

adrenergic symptoms—Symptoms, including sweating and heart palpitations, that occur when low blood glucose levels trigger the release of the hormone epinephrine into the blood.

alpha-glucosidase inhibitors—Oral diabetes drugs that lower the peak levels of blood glucose and insulin after a meal. They act by inhibiting intestinal enzymes that digest complex carbohydrates and sucrose, delaying the absorption of carbohydrates. Examples are acarbose (Precose) and miglitol (Glyset).

antioxidants—Substances that help the body neutralize free radicals, which can cause cell damage. Naturally occurring antioxidants include beta-carotene, vitamin C, vitamin E, and selenium.

atherosclerosis—An accumulation of deposits of fat and fibrous tissue, called plaques, within the walls of arteries that can narrow these blood vessels and reduce blood flow.

autonomic neuropathy—Damage to nerves that control involuntary actions in the body, such as digestion, heart rate, and blood pressure.

biguanides—Oral diabetes drugs that decrease glucose production by the liver and increase glucose uptake by cells. Do not cause hypoglycemia when used alone. Metformin (Glucophage, Glucophage XR) is the only available biguanide.

blood osmolarity—The thickness of the blood. High blood glucose increases blood osmolarity.

cardiovascular disease—Disease affecting the arteries that supply blood to the heart and other organs. Coronary heart disease, stroke, and peripheral vascular disease are the most common types of cardiovascular disease.

cataract—A cloudiness or opacification of the lens of the eye that can lead to visual impairment.

coronary heart disease—A narrowing of the arteries that supply blood to the heart. Caused by atherosclerosis. Can reduce or completely block blood flow to the heart. Also called coronary artery disease.

diabetic foot ulcer—An open sore on the foot that occurs in people with diabetes who have damage to nerves and/or poor blood flow to the feet.

diabetic ketoacidosis—An acute complication of diabetes (usually type 1) that results from a nearly complete lack of insulin. The body is forced to use fatty acids instead of glucose as a major source of energy. The resulting breakdown of fatty acids to ketone bodies raises the acidity of the blood to dangerous levels. Symptoms include nausea, vomiting, heavy breathing, dry or flushed skin, and fruity breath.

diuretics—Drugs that increase urine production by enhancing loss of sodium through the kidneys. They are used to eliminate excess fluid from the body and to treat high blood pressure.

D-phenylalanine derivatives—Oral diabetes drugs that stimulate rapid insulin secretion to reduce the rise in blood glucose that occurs soon after eating. The only such drug available is nateglinide (Starlix).

external insulin pump—A pump, usually worn on a belt, that delivers a continuous flow of insulin along with added amounts before meals through a needle inserted under the skin of the abdomen, thigh, or buttocks.

fasting blood glucose test—Measures blood glucose levels after an overnight fast. Diabetes is diagnosed if blood glucose is above 125 mg/dL on at least two tests.

free radicals—Chemical compounds that can damage cells and oxidize low density lipoproteins, making them more likely to be deposited in the walls of arteries.

gestational diabetes—A type of diabetes that occurs during pregnancy. About 2% to 5% of pregnant women develop the condition, which usually goes away when the pregnancy is over. It signals a high risk of type 2 diabetes later in life.

glaucoma—An eye disease characterized by damage to the optic nerve. Increased pressure within the eyeball is a risk factor.

glucagon—A hormone that raises blood glucose levels by signaling the liver to convert amino acids and glycogen to glucose, which is then released into the bloodstream. Glucagon may be given by injection to raise blood glucose levels in the case of severe hypoglycemia.

glucose—A simple sugar that circulates in the blood and provides energy to the body. Excess glucose is normally converted to glycogen or triglycerides, mainly in the liver, when there is adequate insulin in the blood.

glucose transport proteins—Proteins that carry glucose from the outside of a cell to the inside.

glycogen—A complex carbohydrate that is stored in the liver and muscles until it is needed for energy.

hemoglobin A1c (HbA1c) test—A test that measures the amount of glucose attached to hemoglobin. The test is routinely used to assess blood glucose control over the previous two to three months.

high density lipoprotein (HDL)—A lipid-carrying protein that protects against atherosclerosis by removing cholesterol deposited in artery walls.

hyperglycemia—High blood glucose levels.

GLOSSARY—continued

hyperosmolar nonketotic state—A medical emergency characterized by extremely high blood glucose levels in people with type 2 diabetes. It is usually caused by the physical stress of an injury or major illness. Symptoms include dry or parched mouth, nausea, vomiting, rapid and shallow breathing, and warm, dry skin.

hypoglycemia—Low blood glucose levels. May be symptomless or may cause symptoms like shaking and sweating. May progress to changes in mental status (confusion, sleepiness) or even coma. Almost always reversed by eating a fast-acting carbohydrate or, if necessary, by injecting glucagon.

implantable insulin pump—A pump, placed under the skin of the abdomen, that delivers insulin through a catheter into the abdominal cavity. It delivers insulin at a constant rate, along with added amounts for meals. The device is still under development and is not yet approved by the U.S. Food and Drug Administration.

insulin—A hormone normally produced by the pancreas that regulates the production of glucose by the liver and the utilization of glucose by cells. Without adequate insulin, glucose accumulates in the blood and causes hyperglycemia, the hallmark of diabetes. Insulin is also a medication taken by people with diabetes whose pancreas does not make enough insulin.

insulin pen—A combined insulin container and needle that makes injection of insulin more convenient.

insulin syringe—A syringe with a needle that is used to inject insulin. The most common way to administer insulin.

intermediate-acting insulin—Insulin medication that begins working in 1 to 4 hours, peaks at 6 to 12 hours, and lasts for about 14 to 24 hours. Examples are NPH insulin and lente insulin.

islets of Langerhans—Cellular masses in the pancreas that contain insulin- and glucagon-secreting cells. Also called pancreatic islets.

jet injector—A needle-free way of injecting insulin that uses a high-pressure jet of air to send a fine stream of insulin through the skin.

ketone bodies—Occur when a nearly complete lack of insulin forces the body to use fatty acids instead of glucose as a source of energy. The accumulation of ketone bodies increases the acidity of the blood to dangerous levels.

laser photocoagulation—A treatment for proliferative retinopathy or macular edema that slows or halts vision loss by destroying diseased blood vessels in the retina.

long-acting insulin—Insulin medication that begins working in 4 to 6 hours, peaks at 18 to 28 hours, and lasts for up to 36 hours. Examples are insulin glargine (Lantus) and ultralente insulin.

low density lipoprotein (LDL)—A protein that transports cholesterol in the blood. A major contributor to atherosclerosis.

macular edema—A swelling of the macula, a small area at the center of the retina of the eye that is responsible for central and fine-detail vision. Swelling is caused by leakage and accumulation of fluid from diseased blood vessels.

meglitinides—Oral diabetes drugs that induce the secretion of insulin by the pancreas dependent on the amount of glucose in the blood. These drugs have a more rapid effect on insulin levels than sulfonylureas. The only approved drug in this class is repaglinide (Prandin).

metabolic syndrome—A condition characterized by a group of findings, including elevated blood glucose levels, high triglycerides, low HDL cholesterol, high blood pressure, and obesity that may be initiated by a genetic predisposition to insulin resistance and an accumulation of fat in the abdomen. Also called syndrome X or insulin resistance syndrome.

microalbuminuria—Small amounts of a protein called albumin in the urine that are a first sign of kidney dysfunction.

mononeuropathy—Nerve damage resulting from disruption of the blood supply to one nerve or nerve group. Leads to the sudden onset of pain or weakness in the area served by the affected nerve or nerve group.

nephropathy—Kidney disease.

neuropathy—Nerve damage. Diabetes can result in three types of neuropathy: peripheral neuropathy, mononeuropathy, and autonomic neuropathy.

oral glucose tolerance test—A test in which a person fasts overnight and then drinks a solution containing 75 g of glucose. Diabetes is diagnosed if two hours later blood glucose is 200 mg/dL or more.

pancreas—An organ, located behind and beneath the lower part of the stomach, that produces and secretes insulin and glucagon. The pancreas also makes digestive juices.

pancreatic islets—see islets of Langerhans

peripheral neuropathy—A slow, progressive loss of function of the sensory nerves in the limbs that causes numbness, tingling, and pain in the legs and hands.

peripheral vascular disease—Atherosclerosis in the arteries leading to the legs and feet.

pre-diabetes—Diagnosed when blood glucose levels are higher than normal but not high enough for a diagnosis of diabetes—that is, a fasting blood glucose level between 110 and 125 mg/dL or a blood glucose level between 140 and 199 mg/dL on an oral glucose tolerance test. Formerly called impaired fasting glucose or impaired glucose tolerance.

rapid-acting insulin—Insulin medication that begins working in 30 minutes to 1 hour, peaks at 2 to 4 hours, and lasts for about 6 to 8 hours. Also called regular insulin or short-acting insulin.

retinopathy—Damage to the retina caused by changes in the tiny blood vessels that supply the retina. Advanced disease may require treatment with a procedure called laser photocoagulation.

statins—Drugs that reduce blood levels of cholesterol by blocking its formation.

sulfonylureas—Oral diabetes drugs that stimulate the pancreas to secrete more insulin. Examples are chlorpropamide (Diabinese) and glyburide (DiaBeta, Glynase, Micronase).

thiazolidinediones—Oral diabetes drugs that increase the sensitivity of cells to insulin. Examples are pioglitazone (Actos) and rosiglitazone (Avandia).

tight glucose control—Achieving near normal levels of blood glucose by monitoring blood glucose several times a day and adjusting doses of insulin or oral diabetes drugs accordingly. Aimed at preventing or slowing the progression of long-term complications of diabetes. Also called intensive glucose control.

type 1 diabetes—An autoimmune disease that destroys the ability of beta cells in the pancreas to make insulin. Occurs most commonly in children and young adults. Daily insulin injections are necessary to stay alive.

type 2 diabetes—The most common type of diabetes; accounts for about 90% to 95% of all cases in the United States. Develops when the pancreas cannot make enough insulin to overcome the body's resistance to insulin action. Occurs most often in overweight or obese people over the age of 40, but its occurrence in overweight children is on the rise.

very rapid-acting insulin—Insulin medication that begins working in about 10 to 20 minutes, peaks at about 2 hours, and lasts for about 4 hours. Examples are insulin aspart (Novolog) and insulin lispro (Humalog).

vitreous humor—A thick, gel-like substance that fills the back of the eyeball behind the lens.

HEALTH INFORMATION ORGANIZATIONS AND SUPPORT GROUPS

American Association of Diabetes Educators
100 West Monroe St., Ste. 400
Chicago, IL 60603-1901
☎ 312-424-2426
www.diabeteseducator.org
Organization of health professionals educating people on diabetes management. Provides referrals to local diabetes educators.

American Diabetes Association
Customer Service
1701 North Beauregard St.
Alexandria, VA 22311
☎ 800-342-2383
www.diabetes.org
National organization that funds research, provides information and publications, and offers referrals to support groups and education classes. Look in the white pages for your local chapter.

American Dietetic Association
120 S. Riverside Plaza, Ste. 2000
Chicago, IL 60606-6995
☎ 800-366-1655/312-899-0040
www.eatright.org
Provides nutrition and weight control information, direct access to a registered dietitian, recorded nutrition messages, and referrals to local dietitians.

Joslin Diabetes Center
One Joslin Pl.
Boston, MA 02215
☎ 617-732-2400
www.joslin.harvard.edu
Diabetes treatment, research, and education center affiliated with Harvard Medical School that has treatment centers nationwide. Also produces publications.

National Diabetes Information Clearinghouse
One Information Way
Bethesda, MD 20892-3560
☎ 800-860-8747/301-654-3327
www.niddk.nih.gov/health/diabetes/ndic.htm
Collects and disseminates information on diabetes, responds to requests for information, and provides publications.

National Institute of Diabetes and Digestive and Kidney Diseases
Office of Communications and Public Liaison
Building 31, Rm. 9A04
31 Center Dr., MSC 2560
Bethesda, MD 20892
☎ 800-891-5390/301-654-4415
www.niddk.nih.gov
Conducts and supports research on diabetes, as well as kidney, metabolic, and endocrine diseases.

National Kidney Foundation
30 East 33rd St., Ste. 1100
New York, NY 10016
☎ 800-622-9010/212-889-2210
www.kidney.org
Health organization working for the prevention, treatment, and cure of kidney disease. Provides information and education on diabetes and kidney disease, as well as on organ donation.

LEADING HOSPITALS FOR ENDOCRINOLOGY

U.S. News & World Report and the National Opinion Research Center, a social-science research group at the University of Chicago, recently conducted their 14th annual nationwide survey of 8,160 physicians in 17 medical specialties. The doctors nominated up to five hospitals they consider best from among 6,003 U.S. hospitals. This is the current list of the 10 best endocrinology hospitals, as determined by the doctors' recommendations from 2001, 2002, and 2003; federal data on death rates; and factual data regarding quality indicators, such as the ratio of registered nurses to patients and the use of advanced technology. Since the results reflect the doctors' opinions, however, they are, to some degree, subjective. Any institution listed is considered a leading center, and the rankings do not imply that other hospitals cannot or do not deliver excellent care.

1. **Mayo Clinic**
   Rochester, MN
   ☎ 507-284-2511
   www.mayoclinic.org

2. **Massachusetts General Hospital**
   Boston, MA
   ☎ 617-726-2000
   www.mgh.harvard.edu

3. **Johns Hopkins Hospital**
   Baltimore, MD
   ☎ 800-507-9952/410-955-5000
   www.hopkinsmedicine.org

4. **University of California, San Francisco Medical Center**
   San Francisco, CA
   ☎ 888-689-UCSF/415-476-1000
   www.ucsfhealth.org

5. **University of Virginia Medical Center**
   Charlottesville, VA
   ☎ 800-251-3627/434-924-3627
   www.med.virginia.edu

6. **Barnes-Jewish Hospital**
   St. Louis, MO
   ☎ 314-747-3000
   www.barnesjewish.org

7. **Brigham and Women's Hospital**
   Boston, MA
   ☎ 617-732-5500
   www.brighamandwomens.org

8. **University of California, Los Angeles Medical Center**
   Los Angeles, CA
   ☎ 800-825-2631/310-825-9111
   www.healthcare.ucla.edu

9. **Beth Israel Deaconess Medical Center**
   Boston, MA
   ☎ 800-896-1048/617-667-7000
   www.bidmc.harvard.edu

10. **New York-Presbyterian Hospital**
    New York, NY
    ☎ 212-305-2500
    www.nyp.org

INSULIN THERAPY FOR TYPE 1 AND TYPE 2 DIABETES

Insulin therapy is required for the treatment of people with type 1 diabetes, and some people with type 2 diabetes need insulin as well. Between 6 and 7 million Americans use insulin. Recent advances, such as the insulin pump and types of insulin that more closely mimic the body's own insulin, have changed the way people with diabetes treat their disease. In the article reprinted here from the *Journal of the American Medical Association,* Dawn E. DeWitt, M.D., M.Sc., and Irl B. Hirsch, M.D., review the results of nearly 100 studies on insulin therapy.

Four main types of insulin are available, and each type has a different onset and duration of action. "Physiologic" insulin therapy attempts to mimic the body's own insulin secretion by providing a constant, low level of insulin in the blood between meals and extra insulin after a meal to remove glucose from the bloodstream. Much research has examined which combination of insulin types—as well as the best insulin-oral medication combination for type 2 diabetes—will provide optimal blood glucose control with the lowest risk of hypoglycemia (dangerously low blood glucose levels). Although insulin therapy has become increasingly complex, the advantage is that treatment can be tailored to a person's specific needs.

Several studies in people with type 1 diabetes have shown that using an intermediate- or long-acting insulin (such as NPH, lente, ultralente, or insulin glargine) once or twice a day, along with a more rapid-acting insulin (such as regular insulin, insulin lispro, or insulin aspart) at each meal, is associated with higher patient satisfaction than conventional twice-a-day injections. A major reason is that this approach allows people to skip meals or to be more flexible about mealtimes without worrying about hypoglycemia. "This approach requires more injections," the reviewers write, "but surveys show that patients with type 1 [diabetes] are injecting insulin more frequently and they prefer the dietary freedom, with education about more complex strategies for their care, rather than simplistic rules."

The search continues for the optimal insulin therapy for people with type 2 diabetes as well. Research shows that 53% of people taking oral medications will need insulin after six years, and nearly 80% after nine years. These patients are often reluctant to begin insulin therapy. The researchers point out that people with type 2 diabetes are generally more satisfied with simpler regimens, fewer injections, and insulin pens or premixed injections. Research has also shown that insulin in combination with metformin is associated with similar blood glucose control but less weight gain and fewer hypoglycemic episodes than a combination of insulin and a sulfonylurea.

The reviewers conclude that "treatment goals and intensity of insulin therapy must be individualized since young patients may benefit the most from intensive therapy and even expensive therapies may be cost-effective, while older patients without complications may not benefit as much from intensive therapy with its attendant risks."

Outpatient Insulin Therapy in Type 1 and Type 2 Diabetes Mellitus

Scientific Review

Dawn E. DeWitt, MD, MSc

Irl B. Hirsch, MD

Context Newer insulin therapies, including the concept of physiologic basal-prandial insulin and the availability of insulin analogues, are changing clinical diabetes care. The key to effective insulin therapy is an understanding of principles that, when implemented, can result in improved diabetes control.

Objective To systematically review the literature regarding insulin use in patients with type 1 and type 2 diabetes mellitus (DM).

Data Sources A MEDLINE search was performed to identify all English-language articles of randomized controlled trials involving insulin use in adults with type 1 or type 2 DM from January 1, 1980, to January 8, 2003. Bibliographies and experts were used to identify additional studies.

Study Selection and Data Extraction Studies were included (199 for type 1 DM and 144 for type 2 DM, and 38 from other sources) if they involved human insulins or insulin analogues, were at least 4 weeks long with at least 10 patients in each group, and glycemic control and hypoglycemia were reported. Studies of insulin-oral combination were similarly selected.

Data Synthesis Twenty-eight studies for type 1 DM, 18 for type 2 DM, and 48 for insulin-oral combination met the selection criteria. In patients with type 1 DM, physiologic replacement, with bedtime basal insulin and a mealtime rapid-acting insulin analogue, results in fewer episodes of hypoglycemia than conventional regimens. Rapid-acting insulin analogues are preferred over regular insulin in patients with type 1 DM since they improve HbA_{1C} and reduce episodes of hypoglycemia. In patients with type 2 DM, adding bedtime neutral protamine Hagedorn (isophane) insulin to oral therapy significantly improves glycemic control, especially when started early in the course of disease. Bedtime use of insulin glargine results in fewer episodes of nighttime hypoglycemia than neutral protamine Hagedorn regimens. For patients with more severe insulin deficiency, a physiologic insulin regimen should allow lower glycemic targets in the majority of patients. Adverse events associated with insulin therapy include hypoglycemia, weight gain, and worsening diabetic retinopathy if hemoglobin A_{1C} levels decrease rapidly.

Conclusions Many options for insulin therapy are now available. Physiologic insulin therapy with insulin analogues is now relatively simple to use and is associated with fewer episodes of hypoglycemia.

JAMA. 2003;289:2254-2264 www.jama.com

Primary care physicians provide diabetes care for 39% of the 16 million patients in the United States (US) with type 1 diabetes mellitus (DM) and 82% of patients with type 2 DM.[1] The greatest change in diabetes therapy in the last decade has been the introduction of insulin analogues. Currently, 6 to 7 million Americans use human insulin or insulin analogues. The availability of the new insulin analogues makes physiologic insulin therapy realistic for many patients, because the onset and duration of the action of these analogues more closely mimic human insulin secretion, thus simplifying insulin dosing and adjustment and increasing flexibility for patients. The use of physiologic insulin replacement and continuous subcutaneous insulin infusion (CSII, or pump therapy) are increasingly popular and have become the criterion standard, with more than 200 000 patients with type 1 DM using CSII therapy worldwide.[2]

The American Diabetes Association recommends a hemoglobin (Hb) A_{1C} level less than 7%.[3] Data from 1988-1995[4] show that 43% of US patients had an HbA_{1C} level greater than 8.0%, 18% had poor control with an HbA_{1C} level greater than 9.5% (24% of the insulin-treated patients had poor control). More than 50% of US patients with type 1 DM

Author Affiliations: Division of General Internal Medicine, Department of Medicine, University of Washington (Dr DeWitt); and Division of Metabolism, Endocrinology, and Nutrition, Department of Medicine, University of Washington, and Diabetes Care Center, University of Washington Medical Center (Dr Hirsch), Seattle.

Corresponding Author and Reprints: Dawn E. DeWitt, MD, MSc, Rural Clinical School, University of Melbourne, PO Box 6500, Shepparton VIC 3632, Australia (e-mail: ddewitt@unimelb.edu.au).

Scientific Review and Clinical Applications Section Editor: Wendy Levinson, MD, Contributing Editor. We encourage authors to submit papers to "Scientific Review and Clinical Applications." Please contact Wendy Levinson, MD, Contributing Editor, *JAMA*; phone: 312-464-5204; fax: 312-464-5824; e-mail: wendy.levinson@utoronto.ca.

use only 1 to 2 insulin injections per day, a suboptimal, nonphysiologic approach to type 1 DM insulin therapy.[5] Importantly, even many patients with type 2 DM would not achieve adequate control using twice-daily neutral protamine Hagedorn (NPH or isophane insulin).[6]

Most physicians would agree that good diabetes control, which often requires intensive insulin therapy, is desirable for patients with type 1 DM and type 2 DM. Patients receiving intensive therapy with lower HbA_{1C} levels with type 1 DM in the Diabetes Control and Complications Trial, or with type 2 DM in the United Kingdom Prospective Diabetes Study (UKPDS), had fewer, later microvascular complications.[7,8] Interestingly, some data suggest that insulin may benefit patients with DM in other ways. For example, early insulin therapy may preserve β-cell function.[9,10] Insulin therapy can also improve lipid metabolism[11-15] and mortality after myocardial infarction.[16]

With diabetes-related medical costs of $132 billion per year (more than 12% of the US health care budget),[17] many experts question whether intensive insulin therapy (approximately $16 000-30 000 per quality-adjusted life years gained)[17] is cost-effective. In the UKPDS, the incremental yearly cost of intensive insulin therapy for patients with type 2 DM (either with sulfonylurea [SU] agents or with insulin) was $1866,[18] while in the Kumamoto trial, multiple injection therapy for patients with type 2 DM reduced costs from $31 525 for conventional therapy to $30 310, by decreasing complications.[19]

Table 1. Currently Available Insulin Products*

Insulin†	Onset	Peak	Effective Duration, h	Cost per 10 mL per 100 U/mL‡
Rapid-acting	5-15 min	30-90 min	5	
Lispro (Humalog)				$46
Aspart (NovoLog)				$58
Short-acting	30-60 min	2-3 h	5-8	
Regular U100				$25
Regular U500 (concentrated)				$220/20 mL
Buffered regular (Velosulin)				$55
Intermediate-acting				
Isophane insulin (NPH, Humulin N/Novolin N)	2-4 h	4-10 h	10-16	$24-$26
Insulin zinc (Lente, Humulin L/Novolin L)	2-4 h	4-12 h	12-18	$24-$26
Long-acting				
Insulin zinc extended (Ultralente, Humulin U)	6-10 h	10-16 h	18-24	$25
Glargine (Lantus)	2-4 h§	No peak	20-24	$46
Premixed				
70% NPH/30% regular (Humulin 70/30)	30-60 min	Dual	10-16	$25
50% NPH/50% regular (Humulin 50/50)	30-60 min	Dual	10-16	$46
75% NPL/25% lispro (Humalog Mix 75/25)	5-15 min	Dual	10-16	$58
70% NP/30% aspart (NovoLog Mix)	5-15 min	Dual	10-16	$59

Abbreviations: L, Lente; NPH, neutral protamine Hagedorn; NPL, insulin lispro protamine (neutral protamine lispro).
*Adapted with permission from *Practical Insulin: A Handbook for Prescribing Providers*, The American Diabetes Association, 2002.[163]
†Assuming 0.1-0.2 U/kg per injection. Onset and duration vary significantly by injection site.
‡Prices are for comparison and may vary widely. Sources of prices are from Drugstore.com (http://www.drugstore.com) or retail ranges from Costco, Safeway, Rite Aid, and Walgreens.
§Time to steady state.

METHODS

We searched MEDLINE for all English-language articles involving insulin use in adults with type 1 DM (n=199) or type 2 DM (n=144) between January 1, 1980, and January 8, 2003. Bibliographies and experts allowed for the identification of additional relevant abstracts (n=3) and studies (n=35). Randomized controlled trials were included (28 for type 1 DM and 18 for type 2 DM) if they compared currently available human insulins, reported glucose measurements and/or rates of hypoglycemic episodes, and were at least 4 weeks long with at least 10 patients in each group. Using similar criteria, randomized controlled trials of insulin-oral agent combination therapy (n=48) were reviewed in detail. Studies with English-language abstracts or those using animal and human insulins were selected if they were included in previously published reviews or meta-analyses and met our other criteria.

The authors reviewed, summarized, and synthesized the data. We found the literature highly problematic because it lacked standardized medication protocols, methods, and end points. A large majority of trials were sponsored by the pharmaceutical industry. Given the paucity of evidence in some areas, we believe that expert clinical diabetes practice is far ahead of clinical trials.

RESULTS

What Are the Major Types of Insulin?

Rapid-Acting Insulin. Insulin lispro and insulin aspart do not self-aggregate in solution as human (regular) insulin does, and these insulins are rapidly absorbed (TABLE 1). Insulin lispro differs from human insulin by an amino acid exchange of lysine and proline at positions 28 and 29. The substitution of aspartic acid for proline at position 28 created insulin aspart. Rapid-acting insulins are most appropriately injected at mealtime as "prandial" insulin (sometimes referred to as "bolus" insulin) or used in insulin pumps.

Short-Acting Insulin. Regular insulin has a delay to onset of action of 30 to 60 minutes (Table 1). Patients are instructed to inject regular insulin 20 to 30 minutes prior to meals (ie, lag time is the time between injecting insulin and eating) to match insulin availability and carbohydrate absorption. Regular insulin acts almost immediately when injected intravenously.

Intermediate-Acting Insulin. Neutral protamine Hagedorn (isophane insulin; NPH) insulin is slowly absorbed due to the addition of protamine to regular insulin (Table 1). Regular insulin bound to zinc, Lente insulin, has a slightly longer effective duration than

NPH. Lente and NPH are commonly used as twice-daily basal insulins. Neutral protamine lispro (insulin lispro protamine; NPL) and protamine crystalline (crystal) aspart, available in the United States only in premixed insulins, are functionally identical to NPH.

Long-Acting Insulin. Ultralente insulin (insulin zinc extended) is absorbed slowly in its zinc crystalline form. Insulin glargine, a modified human insulin that forms a microprecipitate in the subcutaneous tissue, is released slowly with a peakless delivery of about 20 to 24 hours in most patients (Table 1).

What Are the Major Adverse Effects of Insulin?

Hypoglycemia is the most common adverse effect of insulin therapy. In the Diabetes Control and Complications Trial (type 1 DM),[20] intensive therapy increased the risk of severe hypoglycemia, defined as needing the assistance of another person. Severe hypoglycemia was reported by 26% of patients with a mean of 1.9 episodes per patient per year, and 43% of episodes occurred nocturnally. In the UKPDS, patients with type 2 DM receiving insulin therapy had lower HbA_{1C} levels, but 1% to 2% more patients receiving insulin reported at least 1 episode of severe hypoglycemia per year than those patients receiving other therapies. Intensive therapy, with oral medications or insulin, has been shown to increase the risk of episodes of hypoglycemia.[8]

Generally, patients receiving insulin gain weight. As patients attempt better glycemic control, decreased glycosuria and intermittent overinsulinization can result in hypoglycemia, hunger, and increased caloric intake. In the Diabetes Control and Complications Trial, patients with type 1 DM receiving intensive insulin therapy gained 4.75 kg more than patients receiving conventional therapy during the 3.5- to 9-year study period ($P<.001$), although waist-hip ratios did not differ between groups.[21] In the UKPDS, patients with type 2 DM receiving intensive insulin therapy gained significantly more weight (1.4-2.3 kg) than those patients treated with SUs or metformin.[8] Bedtime administration of NPH produces less weight gain than daytime NPH, making bedtime administration a preferred strategy when starting insulin therapy in patients with type 2 DM.[22,23] In one study, patients gained less weight with insulin glargine than with conventional therapy with NPH.[24]

Rapid improvement in diabetes control results in progressive worsening of retinopathy in approximately 5% of patients.[25-27] Patients with proliferative retinopathy and who have an HbA_{1C} level greater than 10% are at highest risk of worsening retinopathy.[28] In these patients, we recommend reducing the HbA_{1C} level slowly (2% each year) with frequent ophthalmologic examinations (eg, every 6 months or for any symptoms) to ensure aggressive treatment of progressive retinopathy.

What Are the Major Issues Regarding Insulin Delivery?

When prescribing insulin for patients, important issues include insulin pharmacokinetics and compatibility, technological issues, and costs. Insulin absorption variability is the biggest confounder of efforts to mimic physiologic insulin secretion. The onset and duration of action of types of insulin vary greatly when different insulins are mixed, by injection site, and among patients.[29] Large doses of human insulins form an insulin depot, unpredictably prolonging the duration of action; this response is less of an issue for the insulin analogues.[30] Thus, patients injecting 40 U of NPH insulin into their abdominal region before breakfast may have a significantly different onset and peak of action than the same patients injecting 20 U of NPH in their thigh in the evening; mixing insulin lispro with the morning NPH dose and regular with the evening NPH dose would result in further variation. Insulin glargine may not be mixed with other insulins. Cloudy insulins, for example NPH, must be resuspended before administration, and if done improperly the insulin concentration may vary significantly.[31] Importantly, any strategy that increases the consistency of delivery should decrease glucose fluctuations.

Insulin pens are convenient and may help avoid some insulin errors, but insulin cartridges for pens are more expensive than insulin in vials. Patients using insulin pumps must attend to tubing and injection site issues, must closely monitor their blood glucose level, and should have a back-up method of insulin administration.

What Are the Differences Between Physiologic and Nonphysiologic Insulin Regimens?

We refer to regimens that do not mimic normal β-cell secretion as "nonphysiologic insulin replacement" (FIGURE 1). "Physiologic insulin replacement" attempts to mimic normal insulin secretion. In general, physiologic regimens replace basal and prandial insulin (often referred to as "bolus") separately. In our experience, physicians and patients frequently misunderstand this key difference.

Traditionally, NPH was the primary basal insulin and regular was the primary prandial insulin. However, as typically used, each provides both basal and prandial effects. In conventional twice-daily NPH and regular insulin regimens (FIGURE 2), morning regular insulin is responsible for glucose disposal for breakfast, but its effective duration of 5 to 8 hours also makes it prandial insulin at lunch. After the absorption of breakfast (carbohydrate disposal is usually complete by midmorning), the regular insulin becomes, by definition, basal insulin. The morning NPH insulin is basal insulin after breakfast and lunch absorption are complete, and becomes the primary prandial insulin for lunch. But the relatively quick onset of NPH makes it functionally a component of the breakfast prandial insulin. This regimen requires strict consistency of the timing of injections and meals. Delaying lunch frequently results in hypoglycemia, at least for many patients trying to achieve meticulous glycemic control. Because NPH and regular insulin overlap in the later part

Figure 1. Examples of Nonphysiologic Insulin Replacement

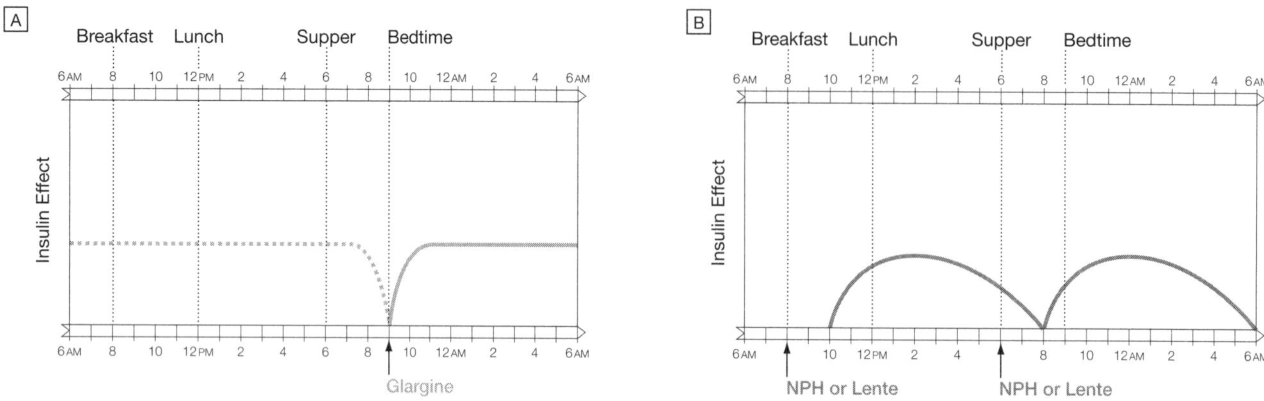

Nonphysiologic insulin replacement does not mimic normal β-cell insulin secretion. A, Once-daily, long-acting insulin glargine is released with a peakless delivery of approximately 20 to 24 hours in most patients. Glargine achieves steady state at approximately 2 hours. Dashed line indicates the effective duration of glargine continuing through the following day. B, Twice-daily, intermediate-acting neutral protamine Hagedorn (isophane insulin; NPH) and Lente (insulin zinc) are commonly used as basal insulin. Arrows indicate insulin injection.

of the morning, many patients require midmorning snacks to prevent hypoglycemia (Figure 2).

Using prandial insulin for each meal (either regular insulin, insulin lispro, or insulin aspart) with separate basal insulin (NPH, Lente, Ultralente, or insulin glargine) adds flexibility to the regimen, and glargine-lispro or glargine-aspart regimens allow patients to skip meals or change mealtimes (FIGURE 3). This approach requires more injections than with conventional twice-daily physiologic regimens, but surveys show that patients with type 1 DM are injecting insulin more frequently and they prefer the dietary freedom, with education about more complex strategies for their care, rather than simplistic rules.[1,32] In one study, 80% of patients preferred a qualitative strategy and 20% preferred a quantitative strategy to a "simple" but relatively inflexible strategy.[33] Dose adjustment is much simpler with true basal-prandial regimens (eg, glargine-lispro) than with insulins that function as both a basal and a prandial insulin (eg, NPH).

Figure 2. Example of Conventional Physiologic Insulin Regimen

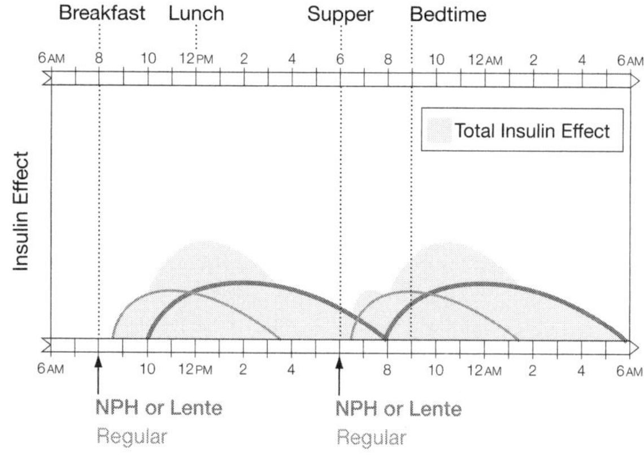

Physiologic insulin replacement with intermediate-acting neutral protamine Hagedorn (isophane insulin; NPH) or Lente (insulin zinc) and short-acting regular insulin (shown in a ratio of 70:30) attempts to mimic normal β-cell insulin secretion. Each insulin serves as both a basal and a prandial insulin. Meal timing and consistency are important for patients using this regimen. Many patients require a midmorning and bedtime snack to prevent hypoglycemia when the effect of the 2 insulins overlap at late morning and nighttime. Moving the dinnertime NPH injection to bedtime decreases the risk of nocturnal hypoglycemia. Arrows indicate insulin injection.

How Does the Patient Use Supplements and Adjustments?

Hyperglycemia correction is an important principle of insulin therapy. A supplement is a predetermined dose of rapid- or short-acting insulin used to correct hyperglycemia. Supplements are easier to determine when basal and prandial insulins are administered separately. Supplements are usually injected with the usual prandial dose of insulin. A conservative dose for patients with type 1 DM is an additional 1 U per 50 mg/dL (2.7 mmol/L) above the target blood glucose level. For patients with type 2 DM, we recommend 1 U of supplemental insulin per 30 mg/dL (1.7 mmol/L) above the target glucose level.

If patients are using insulin supplements between meals, they must beware of "insulin stacking." Injecting additional short- or rapid-acting insulin 1 hour after a dose of regular and NPH insulin would result in insulin stacking and in predictable hypoglycemia within several hours because most of the previously injected insulin has not been ab-

Figure 3. Examples of Physiologic Insulin Delivery Regimen

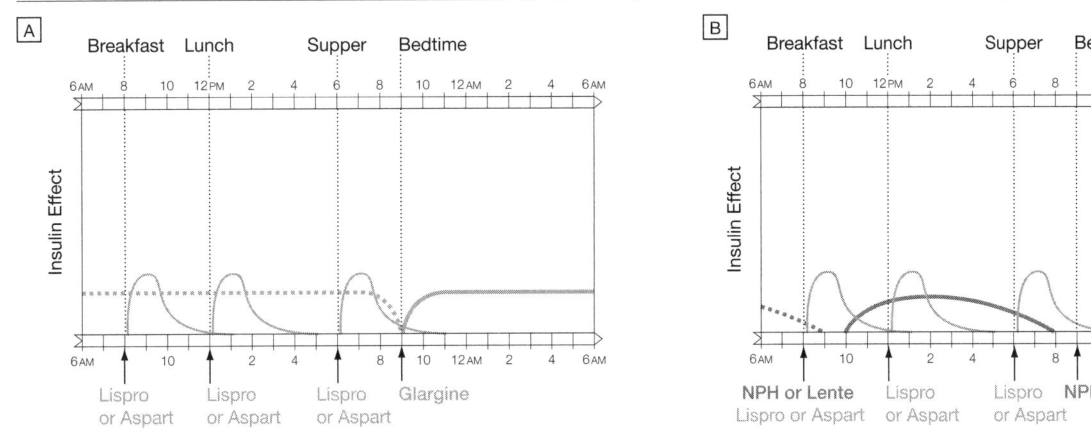

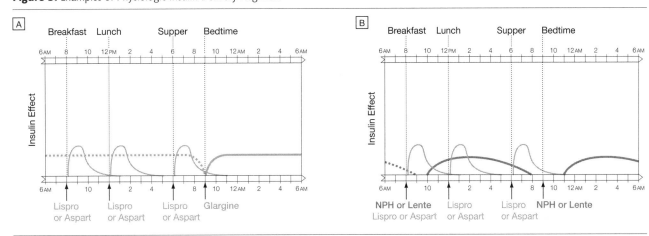

A, Once-daily glargine with lispro or aspart (shown in a ratio of 50:50) allows patients to skip meals or change mealtimes. Insulins lispro and aspart (rapid acting) are prandial insulins and glargine (long acting) is a basal insulin. This regimen is easier to use since it has true basal and prandial insulins. Dashed line indicates the effective duration of glargine continuing through the following day. Glargine achieves steady state at approximately 2 hours. B, Intermediate-acting neutral protamine Hagedorn (isophane insulin; NPH) and Lente (insulin zinc) are basal insulins. Rapid-acting lispro and aspart insulins are prandial insulins. This regimen (shown in a ratio of 50:50) is more difficult to adjust because NPH can act as both a basal and a prandial insulin. Dashed line indicates the effective duration of NPH or Lente continuing through the following day. Arrows indicate insulin injection.

sorbed. If patients are to inject supplements less than 3 hours after a previous insulin dose, they can decrease the supplement by 50%. Patients who exercise may be required to adjust their dose of rapid-acting insulin analogues. Patients who exercise early in the postprandial period (1-3 hours) may need to decrease their dose of rapid-acting insulin by 75%, whereas patients who exercise later in the postprandial period may require a smaller or no change in dose.[34,35]

An "adjustment" means changing the dose of any type of insulin based on a consistent pattern of blood glucose levels. For example, the adjustment for a patient receiving bedtime NPH insulin who has frequent fasting hypoglycemia would be to decrease the bedtime insulin dose. Aggressive but careful adjustments based on patients' injection timing meal patterns and activity levels are key to excellent long-term glucose control.

Why Is It Important for Patients to Self-monitor?

While there is little controversy that all patients receiving insulin should perform self-monitoring of blood glucose tests, there is disagreement about the frequency and timing of the tests. For type 1 DM, the American Diabetes Association suggests 3 or more tests per day.[29] The data are less clear for patients with insulin-requiring type 2 DM. Many type 2 DM studies exclude patients receiving insulin, lump insulin users and nonusers, and were conducted before the availability of insulin analogues and improved self-monitoring of blood glucose equipment. A recent study suggests self-monitoring of blood glucose is associated with improved control in patients with type 2 DM who use the results to adjust insulin doses.[36]

What Regimens Are Best for Patients With Type 1 DM?

Type 1, autoimmune, DM occurs in adults of all ages, including obese patients with phenotypic type 2 DM. Latent autoimmune DM (also known as LADA) of adults can be confused with type 2 DM early in diagnosis, but patients become insulinopenic relatively rapidly.[37]

Nonphysiologic Regimens. Some newly diagnosed patients with type 1 DM or latent autoimmune DM of adults who are still producing endogenous insulin may do well receiving once- or twice-daily basal insulin injections before they progress to complete β-cell failure (Figure 1). The time to complete insulin deficiency varies, but it is generally longer in adults than in children. Even with euglycemia, few physicians would recommend discontinuing insulin completely because intensive insulin therapy appears to promote β-cell preservation.[9,10,38] Data are not available to date to compare different nonphysiologic insulin regimens in this patient population.

Physiologic Regimens (TABLE 2). In patients with severe insulin deficiency, replacement of both prandial and basal insulin components is required. In patients with type 1 DM and no endogenous insulin secretion, it is very difficult to safely reach target HbA_{1C} level (<7%) with conventional insulin therapy, twice-daily NPH, and regular insulin (as shown in Figure 2). This regimen is difficult to adjust, and it is relatively inflexible because it uses both insulin components as both a prandial and a basal insulin. Moving NPH insulin from dinnertime to bedtime was first suggested in the 1980s as a strategy to optimize this conventional regimen.[39] Mixed NPH and regular insulin are given before breakfast, regular insulin is injected before dinner, and NPH is given at bedtime. A recent randomized, crossover study confirmed that this bedtime

Table 2. Available Insulin Delivery Systems and the Cost of a Physiologic Regimen With Each System

Delivery System	Advantages	Disadvantages	Cost (Comparative Examples for Initial and Monthly Cost)* Item	Amount
Syringe	Maximal ability to "freemix" insulin and adjust to patient needs	Multiple injections Need to carry bottles, syringes, and supplies Variable absorption depending on type of insulin and body injection site Lispro and glargine are both clear insulins and therefore difficult to distinguish, patients must read labels carefully	Insulin glargine 1000 U	$44
			Insulin lispro 1000 U	$46
			Syringes for 4 injections/d (120-gauge)	$36
			Total cost per month for glargine at bedtime + lispro 3 times/d	$126 Bedtime NPH + 3 times/d of prandial regular = $25 + $25 + $36 = $86
Pen	Convenient, less to carry Easy to distinguish between insulins by pen color/size Improves dosing accuracy Although not recommended, many use 1 needle per 24 h	For injection, approximately 30% more expensive per 1000 U than bottled insulin	Pen injector	Novopen 3 = $29-$32 retail
			Pen cartridges for 1000 U	NPH = $42 Glargine = $63 Lispro = $63
			Total cost per month for bedtime dose with needles	NPH/prandial lispro = $105 Glargine/lispro = $126
Pump	Fewer injections Physiologic delivery with best glycemic control and fewest hypoglycemic events overall Eliminates variable injection-site absorption	Expensive Additional training needed Patient must be aware of potential technical problems	Pump: Medtronic MiniMed	$5500/60 mo at $92 per month (assumes pump life of 5 years)
			Monthly cost of tubing/reservoirs	$150
			Insulin lispro 2000 U	$92
			Total cost per month	$334

Abbreviation: NPH, neutral protamine Hagedorn (isophane insulin).
*We estimated costs based on 0.9 U/kg for a 70-kg person at 63 U/d, 32 U of each per day, equals 1000 U/mo of each insulin type. Patients are told to discard their unused bottles at the end of the month if they use less insulin.

NPH strategy reduces both HbA_{1C} levels and nocturnal hypoglycemic episodes in patients with type 1 DM.[40]

Overall, patients using insulin analogues (lispro, aspart, glargine) in physiologic regimens (Figure 3A), including patients with hypoglycemia unawareness, have fewer hypoglycemic episodes than patients using traditional insulins (regular and NPH).[41-46] Because of shorter duration of action, insulin lispro (introduced in the United States in 1996) and insulin aspart are only used as prandial insulins or in CSII programs. When patients use insulins lispro or aspart, they have fewer episodes of severe hypoglycemia and nocturnal hypoglycemia than with regular insulin[47-50] (eTABLE 1[42-44,46,50-72] and eTABLE 2[12,24,27,41,53-67,72-83]; tables are published online at http://www.jama.com). Lag time depends on the onset of action of the prandial insulin used (eg, 30 minutes for regular insulin and none for insulin lispro or aspart). An inadequate lag time results in postprandial hyperglycemia and in later risk of hypoglycemia. Patient compliance with the recommended 30-minute lag time for regular insulin is 30% to 70% (patients inject insulin closer to or at mealtime.[84,85] The lack of required lag time for rapid-acting insulins and improved matching of action with carbohydrate absorption explain their clinical advantage (Figure 3).

Data on regimens using rapid-acting analogues with basal NPH are mixed (Figure 3B). Improvements in HbA_{1C} levels have not been seen when analogues are given with basal NPH provided once or twice daily, because the improvement in postprandial hyperglycemia seen with the rapid-acting analogues is negated by higher preprandial and overnight glycemia (compared with regular insulin). One study using small doses of NPH given with insulin lispro before each meal and at bedtime, to better control basal needs between meals, showed decreased HbA_{1C} levels and episodes of hypoglycemia.[62] However, in a recent study of patients with type 1 DM receiving NPH basal insulin (1-2 injections per day) with prandial lispro, adding an additional injection of NPH at lunchtime in an attempt to give smoother basal control resulted in 6.9 more episodes of severe hypoglycemia per patient-year ($P = .007$).[86] Ultralente, which is longer acting than NPH or Lente, was developed to improve basal insulin delivery. However, twice-daily Ultralente, as compared with Lente, mildly improves fasting glucose levels but increases episodes of hypoglycemia.[87]

Insulin glargine became available in the United States in 2001. Theoretically, this peakless, long-acting basal insulin analogue should reduce hypoglycemia and improve glycemic control.[88] In actuality, reductions in episodes of hypoglycemia, especially nocturnal hypoglycemia, occur consistently whereas reductions in HbA_{1C} levels have been more difficult to achieve (eTables 1 and 2; tables are published online at http://www.jama.com). A large multicenter trial of patients with type 1 DM using insulin glargine with prandial regular insulin showed no change in HbA_{1C} levels, although 25% fewer hypoglycemic episodes were noted.[42] When insulin lispro was used as the prandial insulin, no differences in HbA_{1C} levels or hypoglycemic epsisodes were observed, but patients receiving glargine gained slightly less weight.[63] When glargine and lispro were compared with NPH and regular insulin in adoles-

Figure 4. Progressive Decline in β-Cell Function and Insulin Secretion in Type 2 Diabetes Mellitus

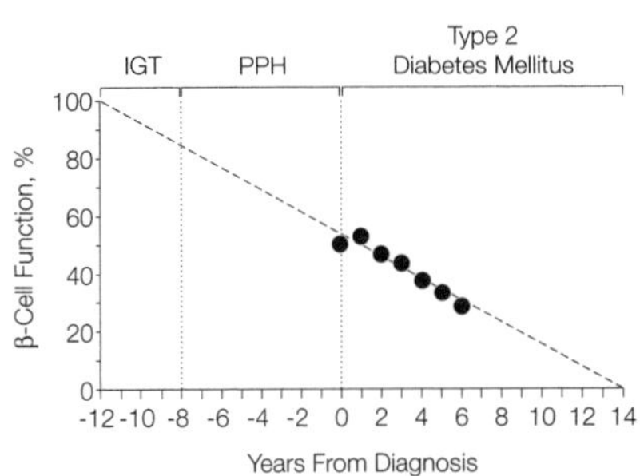

Data show 50% of normal β-cell function at diagnosis of type 2 diabetes mellitus (year 0) and a steady decline up to 6 years following diagnosis. Clinically, most patients have had prediabetes (impaired glucose tolerance [IGT] and postprandial hyperglycemia [PPH]) for some time before clinical diagnosis of type 2 diabetes mellitus. Dotted line shows the extrapolation of β-cell function before and after diagnosis of diabetes. Adapted with permission from *Diabetes Reviews*[133] based on data from the United Kingdom Prospective Diabetes Study.[92]

cents, results of HbA_{1C} levels were similar, but the glargine-lispro regimen produced fewer hypoglycemic episodes.[61] However, in a population with a lower baseline HbA_{1C} level (7.1%), substituting insulin glargine for NPH, with prandial insulin lispro, decreased hypoglycemic episodes and HbA_{1C} levels.[89]

It may be that the main impact of physiologic insulin regimens and insulin glargine in particular is that the separation of prandial and basal components improves our understanding of insulin use, simplifies dosing adjustments, and allows patients more flexibility in meal timing. With a distinctly different basal insulin component (glargine or pump therapy), patients need approximately half of their insulin as basal insulin. When initiating a basal-prandial regimen, patients should decrease the calculated 50% basal insulin dose by 20% to avoid hypoglycemia. Using this calculation, one third of patients are receiving the correct dose, one third need more, and one third need less basal insulin.[90]

When Should Insulin Be Used in Type 2 DM?

Most patients with type 2 DM will eventually need insulin. Insulin therapy was started in patients with type 2 DM with a mean HbA_{1C} level of 10.4% in the United States,[91] and the UKPDS[92] showed that β-cell failure is progressive; 50% of normal β-cell function at diagnosis with a steady decline following diagnosis (FIGURE 4). Concomitantly, 53% of patients with type 2 DM initially treated with SUs required insulin therapy by 6 years, and almost 80% required insulin by 9 years.[93,94] Although we may be diagnosing DM earlier and thus altering this time frame, physicians should consider starting insulin therapy in patients whose HbA_{1C} level approaches 8% despite optimal oral therapy.

Improved glycemic control delays or prevents complications in patients with type 2 DM,[8,95,96] although patients often need an insulin dosage of greater than 100 U/d to achieve glycemic control.[94] Patients with type 2 DM often resist physician recommendations to start insulin therapy, partly because of misperceptions that starting insulin means the patient and physician have failed. Several unmasked studies suggest that switching from oral agents to the use of insulin in patients with type 2 DM improves treatment satisfaction, general well being, and quality of life, especially if patients previously had poor glycemic control.[22,75,79,97] When choosing an insulin regimen, the benefits of intensive therapy must be tempered by cost and ease of regimen. In general, treatment satisfaction is better with simpler regimens. Patients allocated to strict control (fasting plasma glucose level <117 mg/dL [6.5 mmol/L]) or less strict control (fasting plasma glucose level <153 mg/dL [8.5 mmol/L]) for 1 year reported improved mood and general well being if their HbA_{1C} level decreased 1% or more, but strict targets increased perceived treatment burden.[98] It has been shown that patients prefer insulin glargine to NPH,[66] twice-daily NPH to Ultralente, and insulin pen administration or premixed insulin to free-mixed insulin administered with syringes.[99-103]

What Is the Best Regimen for Patients With Type 2 DM?

Combination Oral Agent/Insulin Therapy. When using bedtime basal insulin (NPH or glargine), continuing 1 or 2 daytime oral medications is reasonable (**eTABLE 3**[6,8,15,94,97,104-132,134-146]; table is published online at http://www.jama.com). Metformin with insulin results in similar metabolic control, less weight gain, lower insulin doses, and fewer hypoglycemic episodes than insulin alone or insulin/SU therapy.* Thus, metformin and insulin may be the best combination for the majority of patients with type 2 DM who do not have contraindications. However, it should be emphasized that the goal is the target HbA_{1C} level, not lower insulin dose. Patients who must discontinue metformin because of increasing plasma creatinine levels should have their insulin dose increased 20% to 36% to maintain glycemic control.[147]

Combining SUs with insulin lowers insulin doses (25%-50%) with less weight gain, but increases cost.† Sulfonylureas increase endogenous insulin secretion (C-peptide) early in the disease process. Improvement of HbA_{1C} with SU use in the UKPDS was in patients whose HbA_{1C} levels were well below 10%.[93] As insulin production declines and HbA_{1C} levels approach 10%, the combination of insulin and SUs eventually becomes ineffective.[149]

Insulin secretagogues include the SUs and the glinides. Glinides are functionally short-acting SUs and may improve prandial control with or without basal insulin. Not enough data are available to date to endorse their use,[150] especially given their cost, although they may be beneficial in patients with hypoglycemia or who skip meals.

Although thiazolidinediones (TZDs) are effective insulin sensitizers, combined TZD/insulin therapy has been problematic, and TZDs are expensive. Troglitazone was taken off the market due to liver failure, but one randomized trial comparing intensive insulin monotherapy vs insulin with either metformin or troglitazone showed that all therapies lowered HbA_{1C} levels effectively.[151] Patients gained about 4.4 kg while receiv-

*References 97, 113, 114, 119, 120, 140, 144.
†References 105, 110, 119, 123-125, 127, 148.

ing insulin or insulin/troglitazone, but only 0.5 kg while receiving insulin/metformin. Troglitazone significantly reduced the dose of insulin but caused the same rate of hypoglycemic episodes as insulin (2 per month), while patients receiving insulin/metformin reported no hypoglycemia. Pioglitazone and rosiglitazone should not be used with patients in New York Heart Association (NYHA) class III or IV heart failure, and patients' liver function must be monitored. Significant weight gain, pulmonary edema, and heart failure are increasingly associated with TZDs.[152] Given these issues, combination TZD/insulin therapy should be used with caution.

Insulin Therapy. The goals of insulin therapy in both type 1 and type 2 DM are to reach the target HbA_{1C} level with a low rate of hypoglycemic episodes and the least amount of weight gain (eTable 2; table is published online at http://www.jama.com). However, goals must be individualized since older patients with type 2 DM and with no complications may not benefit from intensive therapy. When starting insulin therapy in patients continuing daytime insulin secretagogues or metformin, with an HbA_{1C} level less than 9.5% to 10%, bedtime basal insulin therapy is effective, convenient, and produces less weight gain.[22,23,73] Compared with NPH, basal insulin glargine is associated with 25% fewer nocturnal hypoglycemic episodes, better postdinner control, and slightly less weight gain at twice the cost.[24,41] Both NPH and glargine are easily adjusted based on fasting blood glucose levels. Once-daily Ultralente insulin produces more hypoglycemic episodes than twice-daily NPH despite a higher HbA_{1C} level.[75] If nocturnal hypoglycemia is an issue and glargine is not an option, prandial lispro with SU lowers HbA_{1C} levels with fewer hypoglycemic episodes than NPH with SU.[146]

With progressive β-cell exhaustion, patients will be more successful in achieving glycemic control with progressively more physiologic regimens. Premixed insulins, given twice daily, (70% NPH/30% regular [70N/30R], 70% NP [neutral protamine]/30% aspart [A] [BIAsp], and 75% NPL/25% lispro [L]) are convenient but no prandial insulin is given for lunchtime. BIAsp improves postbreakfast/dinner blood glucose levels, but not HbA_{1C} levels, and decreases severe hypoglycemic episodes by 50% when compared with 70N/30R. Patients who are uncontrolled (ie, not achieving glycemic control) receiving premixed insulin regimens can often achieve control at the same insulin dose by adding lunchtime prandial insulin and by decreasing the morning insulin accordingly. Prandial insulin lispro is associated with fewer episodes of nocturnal hypoglycemia than regular insulin.[82] Another trial of lispro vs regular, with twice-daily basal Lente or Ultralente, showed a lower HbA_{1C} level with lispro at similar insulin doses.[67] Prandial therapy with lispro vs bedtime therapy with NPH lowers HbA_{1C} levels without additional hyperglycemia.[81] Importantly, patients with type 2 DM may require large insulin doses (>1 U/kg) to reach an HbA_{1C} level less than 7%.[6,153,154]

What Are the Advantages of Insulin Pump Therapy?

Patients with type 1 DM receiving CSII therapy show more improvement in HbA_{1C} levels than patients receiving intensive multiple injection therapy[155]; but it remains to be seen whether CSII will reduce the risk of microvascular complications. Compared with multiple injection therapy, CSII reduces hypoglycemic events up to 74%.[155] Intensive insulin therapy reduces costs by decreasing complications; and a study of CSII vs multiple injection therapy in peripartum patients with type 1 DM shows equal costs, but patients preferred pump therapy.[156]

An external pump is programmed to deliver individualized basal rates of short- or rapid-acting insulin (usually 0.5-1.5 U/h). Since patients receiving CSII need less insulin, it has been recommended to decrease the total daily dose by 20% to 30% and then use 50% of that reduced dose as basal insulin.[2] Prandial (bolus) insulin is given by manual activation. Rapid-acting insulins have been shown to be superior to regular insulin in a CSII program because of improved prandial control.[52,70]

The main indications for pump use in patients with type 2 DM without significant C-peptide secretion are severe hypoglycemia and wide fluctuations of glucose levels.[27,80] However, physiologic regimens with insulin glargine and lispro or aspart probably offer the same benefits at lower cost, albeit with more injections.

What Other Approaches Improve Outcomes or Reduce Costs?

While the practice of diabetes care is now increasingly precise, the complexities of care and compliance issues are overwhelming for many physicians. Improving systems of diabetes care may improve glycemic control compared with standard care as shown by (1) frequent insulin dose adjustment by nurse educators via telephone lowered the HbA_{1C} level from 9.4% to 7.8% (0.3% more than standard care)[157]; (2) "telecare" (transmitted data and telephone advice) improved HbA_{1C} levels 1% (vs 1.2%) and saved patients considerable travel time[158]; and (3) using computer decision models for adjustments of insulin doses lowered HbA_{1C} levels approximately 12% and decreased the rate of hypoglycemic episodes by 50% per week.[159,160]

COMMENT

An HbA_{1C} level less than 7% consistently reduces microvascular complications and is now the goal for most patients. Limited data suggest that reducing complications also reduces costs. A team approach with diabetes educators may be more effective at reducing complications at a similar cost. The lack of resources for efficient team care is a major barrier to diabetes care, especially in the primary care community.

Patients with type 1 DM almost always require multiple injections to attain an HbA_{1C} level less than 7%. Physiologic basal-prandial regimens are easier to use and adjust and cause fewer episodes of hypoglycemia. They also provide patients with more flexibility, and studies on patient satisfaction support their use. However, insulin analogues cost 50% more than human insulins.

Patients with type 2 DM who still secrete endogenous insulin often do well receiving oral agents. The choice of oral agent depends largely on adverse effects and cost.[161] Oral agents alone lower HbA_{1C} levels 1% to 2%. Adding bedtime insulin, usually NPH, to oral agents is the standard approach to starting insulin therapy. Although insulin may be added to any approved oral agent, metformin does not cause weight gain and may offer additional cardioprotection[162] and thus is our first choice for use with insulin in patients without contraindications. Oral agents lower the required insulin dose. When patients with type 2 DM become insulin deficient, the principles of insulin use are the same as for patients with type 1 DM. Importantly, patients with type 2 DM often require large insulin doses, for example, 1 to 2 U/kg per day, and the use of lower doses in clinical practice is a common barrier to effective diabetes control.

Finally, treatment goals and intensity of insulin therapy must be individualized since young patients may benefit the most from intensive therapy and even expensive therapies may be cost-effective, while older patients without complications may not benefit as much from intensive therapy with its' attendant risks.

Funding/Support: Dr Hirsch received honoraria for consulting and is on the Speaker's Bureau for Eli Lilly, NovoNordisk, Aventis, and Medtronic MiniMed. He has received grant support from NovoNordisk, Pfizer, and Aventis for clinical trials.
Acknowledgment: We thank Jon Sonoda, RPh, CDE, Pharm D, clinical pharmacist at the Diabetes Care Center, University of Washington Medical Center, for help with obtaining prices for insulin and delivery systems and David Dugdale, MD, for his comments on the manuscript.

REFERENCES

1. Roper ASW. *U. S. Diabetes Patient Market Study*. By permission of East Hanover, NJ: Market Measures/Cozint, an NOP World Co; 2002.
2. Bode BW, Sabbah HT, Gross TM, Fredrickson LP, Davidson PC. Diabetes management in the new millennium using insulin pump therapy. *Diabetes Metab Res Rev*. 2002;18(suppl 1):S14-S20.
3. American Diabetes Association. Clinical practice recommendations 2002. *Diabetes Care*. 2002;25(suppl 1):S1-S147.
4. Saaddine JB, Engelgau MM, Beckless GL, Gregg EW, Thompson TJ, Narayan KM. A diabetes report card for the United States: quality of care in the 1990s. *Ann Intern Med*. 2002;136:565-574.
5. Tabak AG, Tamas G, Zgibor J, et al. Targets and reality. *Diabetes Care*. 2000;23:1284-1289.
6. Abraira C, Henderson WG, Colwell JA, et al. Response to intensive therapy steps and to glipizide dose in combination with insulin in type 2 diabetes. *Diabetes Care*. 1998;21:574-579.
7. Effect of intensive therapy on residual beta-cell function in patients with type 1 diabetes in the diabetes control and complications trial. *Ann Intern Med*. 1998;128:517-523.
8. Intensive blood-glucose control with sulfonylureas or insulin compared with conventional treatment and risk of complications in patients with type 2 diabetes (UKPDS 33). *Lancet*. 1998;352:837-853.
9. Juneja R, Hirsch IB, Naik RG, et al. Islet cell antibodies and glutamic acid decarboxylase antibodies, but not the clinical phenotype, help to identify type 1(1/2) diabetes in patients presenting with type 2 diabetes. *Metabolism*. 2001;50:1008-1013.
10. Linn T, Ortac K, Laube H, Federlin K. Intensive therapy in adult insulin-dependent diabetes mellitus is associated with improved insulin sensitivity and reserve. *Metabolism*. 1996;45:1508-1513.
11. Rodier M, Colette C, Gouzes C, Michel F, Crastes de Paulet A, Monnier L. Effects of insulin therapy upon plasma lipid fatty acids and platelet aggregation in NIDDM with secondary failure to oral antidiabetic agents. *Diabetes Res Clin Pract*. 1995;28:19-28.
12. Landstedt-Hallin L, Adamson U, Arner P, Bolinder J, Lins PE. Comparison of bedtime NPH or preprandial regular insulin combined with glibenclamide in secondary sulfonylurea failure. *Diabetes Care*. 1995;18:1183-1186.
13. Rivellese AA, Patti L, Romano E, et al. Effect of insulin and sulfonylurea therapy, at the same level of blood glucose control, on low density lipoprotein subfractions in type 2 diabetic patients. *J Clin Endocrinol Metab*. 2000;85:4188-4192.
14. Romano G, Patti L, Innelli F, et al. Insulin and sulfonylurea therapy in NIDDM patients. *Diabetes*. 1997;46:1601-1606.
15. Wolffenbuttel BH, Weber RF, van Koetsveld PM, Weeks L, Verschoor L. A randomized crossover study of sulfonylurea and insulin treatment in patients with type 2 diabetes poorly controlled on dietary therapy. *Diabet Med*. 1989;6:520-525.
16. Malmberg K. Prospective randomised study of intensive insulin treatment on long term survival after acute myocardial infarction in patients with diabetes mellitus. *BMJ*. 1997;314:1512-1515.
17. American Diabetes Association. Economic costs of diabetes in the US in 2002. *Diabetes Care*. 2003;26:917-932.
18. Gray A, Raikou M, McGuire A, et al. Cost effectiveness of an intensive blood glucose control policy in patients with type 2 diabetes. *BMJ*. 2000;320:1373-1378.
19. Wake N, Hisashige A, Katayama T, et al. Cost-effectiveness of intensive insulin therapy for type 2 diabetes. *Diabetes Res Clin Pract*. 2000;48:201-210.
20. Epidemiology of severe hypoglycemia in the diabetes control and complications trial. *Am J Med*. 1991;90:450-459.
21. Influence of intensive diabetes treatment on body weight and composition of adults with type 1 diabetes in the Diabetes Control and Complications Trial. *Diabetes Care*. 2001;24:1711-1721.
22. Yki-Jarvinen H, Kauppala M, Kujansuu E, et al. Comparison of insulin regimens in patients with non-insulin-dependent diabetes mellitus. *N Engl J Med*. 1992;327:1426-1433.
23. Yki-Jarvinen H. Comparison of insulin regimens for patients with type 2 diabetes. *Curr Opin Endocrinol Diabetes*. 2000;7:175-183.
24. Rosenstock J, Schwartz SL, Clark CM Jr, Park GD, Donley DW, Edwards MB. Basal insulin therapy in type 2 diabetes. *Diabetes Care*. 2001;24:631-636.
25. Helve E, Laati Kainen L, Merenmies L, Koivisto VA. Continuous insulin infusion therapy and retinopathy in patients with type I diabetes. *Acta Endocrinol (Copenh)*. 1987;115:313-319.
26. Dahl-Jorgensen K, Brinchmann-Hansen O, Hanssen KF, Sarvik L, Aagenaes O. Rapid tightening of blood glucose control leads to transient deterioration of retinopathy in insulin dependent diabetes mellitus. *BMJ (Clin Res Ed)*. 1985;290:811-815.
27. Jennings AM, Lewis KS, Murdoch S, Talbot JF, Bradley C, Ward JD. Randomized trial comparing continuous subcutaneous insulin infusion and conventional insulin therapy in type II diabetic patients poorly controlled with sulfonylureas. *Diabetes Care*. 1991;14:738-744.
28. Chantelau E, Kohner EM. Why some cases of retinopathy worsen when diabetic control improves. *BMJ*. 1997;315:1105-1106.
29. Insulin administration. *Diabetes Care*. 2000;(23 suppl 1):S86-S89.
30. Galloway JA, Rost MA, Rathmacher RP, Carmichael RH. A comparison of acid regular and neutral regular insulin. *Diabetes*. 1973;22:471-479.
31. Jehle PM, Micheler C, Jehle DR, Breitig D, Boehm BO. Inadequate suspension of neutral protamine Hagedorn (NPH) insulin in pens. *Lancet*. 1999;354:1604-1607.
32. Training in flexible, intensive insulin management to enable dietary freedom in people with type 1 diabetes. *BMJ*. 2002;325:746.
33. Kalergis M, Pacuad D, Strycher I, Meltzer S, Jones PJ, Yale JF. Optimizing insulin delivery. *Diabetes Obes Metab*. 2000;2:299-305.
34. Rabasa-Lhoret R, Bourque J, Ducros F, Chiasson JL. Guidelines for premeal insulin dose reduction for postprandial exercise of different intensities and durations in type 1 diabetic subjects treated intensively with a basal-bolus insulin regimen (ultralente- lispro). *Diabetes Care*. 2001;24:625-630.
35. Tuominen JA, Karonen SL, Malamies L, Bolli G, Koivisto VA. Exercise-induced hypoglycaemia in IDDM patients treated with a short-acting insulin analogue. *Diabetologia*. 1995;38:106-111.
36. Franciosi M, Pellegrini F, De Berardis G, et al. The impact of blood glucose self-monitoring on metabolic control and quality of life in type 2 diabetic patients. *Diabetes Care*. 2001;24:1870-1877.
37. Palmer JP, Hirsch IB. What's in a name. *Diabetes Care*. 2003;26:536-538.
38. The effect of intensive treatment of diabetes on the development and progression of long-term complications in insulin-dependent diabetes mellitus. *N Engl J Med*. 1993;329:977-986.
39. Francis AJ, Home PD, Hanning I, Alberti KG, Tunbridge WM. Intermediate acting insulin given at bedtime. *BMJ (Clin Res Ed)*. 1983;286:1173-1176.
40. Fanelli CG, Pampenelli S, Porcellati F, Rossetti P, Brunetti P, Bolli GB. Administration of neutral protamine Hagedorn insulin at bedtime versus with dinner in type 1 diabetes mellitus to avoid nocturnal hypoglycemia and improve control. *Ann Intern Med*. 2002;136:504-514.
41. Yki-Jarvinen HA, Dressler, Ziemen M. Less nocturnal hypoglycemia and better post-dinner glucose control with bedtime insulin glargine compared with bedtime NPH insulin during insulin combination therapy in type 2 diabetes. *Diabetes Care*. 2000;23:1130-1136.
42. Ratner RE, Hirsch IB, Neifing JL, Garg SK, Mecca TE, Wilson CA. Less hypoglycemia with insulin glargine in intensive insulin therapy for type 1 diabetes. *Diabetes Care*. 2000;23:639-643.
43. Raskin P, Holcombe JH, Tamborlane WV, et al. A comparison of insulin lispro and buffered regular human insulin administered via continuous subcutane-

ous insulin infusion pump. *J Diabetes Complications*. 2001;15:295-300.

44. Pfutzner A, Kustner E, Forst T, et al. Intensive insulin therapy with insulin lispro in patients with type 1 diabetes reduces the frequency of hypoglycemic episodes. *Exp Clin Endocrinol Diabetes*. 1996;104:25-30.

45. Riddle MC, Rosenstock J, and H.S. Group. Treatment to target study. *Diabetes*. 2002;51(suppl 2): A113.

46. Ferguson SC, Strachan MW, James JM, Frier BM. Severe hypoglycaemia in patients with type 1 diabetes and impaired awareness of hypoglycaemia. *Diabetes Metab Res Rev*. 2001;17:285-291.

47. Brunelle BL, Llewelyn J, Anderson JH Jr, Gale EA, Koivisto VA. Meta-analysis of the effect of insulin lispro on severe hypoglycemia in patients with type 1 diabetes. *Diabetes Care*. 1998;21:1726-1731.

48. Heller SR, Amiel SA, Mansell P. Effect of the fast-acting insulin analog lispro on the risk of nocturnal hypoglycemia during intensified insulin therapy. *Diabetes Care*. 1999;22:1607-1611.

49. Holleman F, Schmitt HM, Rottier SR, Rees A, Symanowski S, Anderson JH. Reduced frequency of severe hypoglycemia and coma in well-controlled IDDM patients treated with insulin lispro. *Diabetes Care*. 1997; 20:1827-1832.

50. Home PD, Lindholm A, Riis A. Insulin aspart vs human insulin in the management of long-term blood glucose control in type 1 diabetes mellitus. *Diabet Med*. 2000;17:762-770.

51. Daniels AR, Bruce R, McGregor L. Lispro insulin as premeal therapy in type 1 diabetes. *N Z Med J*. 1997; 110:435-438.

52. Zinman B, et al. Insulin lispro in CSII: results of a double-blind crossover study. *Diabetes*. 1997;46:440-443.

53. Vignati L, Anderson JH Jr, Iversen PW. Efficacy of insulin lispro in combination with NPH human insulin twice per day in patients with insulin-dependent or non-insulin-dependent diabetes mellitus. *Clin Ther*. 1997;19:1408-1421.

54. Del Sindaco P, Ciofetta M, Lalli C, et al. Use of the short-acting insulin analogue lispro in intensive treatment of type 1 diabetes mellitus. *Diabet Med*. 1998; 15:592-600.

55. Home PD, Lindholm A, Hylleberg B, Round P. Improved glycemic control with insulin aspart. *Diabetes Care*. 1998;21:1904-1909.

56. Melki V, Ranard E, Lassmann-Vague V, et al. Improvement of HbA_{1c} and blood glucose stability in IDDM patients treated with lispro insulin analog in external pumps. *Diabetes Care*. 1998;21:977-982.

57. Colombel A, Murat J, Krompf M, Kuchly-Anton B, Charbonnel B. Improvement of blood glucose control in type 1 diabetic patients treated with lispro and multiple NPH injections. *Diabet Med*. 1999;16:319-324.

58. Renner R, Pfutzner A, Trautmann M, Harzar O, Sauter K, Landgraf R. Use of insulin lispro in continuous subcutaneous insulin infusion treatment. *Diabetes Care*. 1999;22:784-788.

59. Gale EA. A randomized, controlled trial comparing insulin lispro with human soluble insulin in patients with type 1 diabetes on intensified insulin therapy. *Diabet Med*. 2000;17:209-214.

60. Annuzzi G, Del Prato S, Arcari R, et al. Preprandial combination of lispro and NPH insulin improves overall blood glucose control in type 1 diabetic patients. *Nutr Metab Cardiovasc Dis*. 2001;11:168-175.

61. Murphy NP, Keane SM, Ong KK, Ford ME, Edge JA, Dunger BD. A randomized cross-over trial comparing insulin glargine plus lispro with NPH insulin plus soluble insulin in adolescents with type 1 diabetes. *Diabetes*. 2002;51(suppl 2):A54.

62. Lalli C, Ciofetta M, Del Sindaco P, et al. Long-term intensive treatment of type 1 diabetes with the short-acting insulin analog lispro in variable combination with NPH insulin at mealtime. *Diabetes Care*. 1999;22:468-477.

63. Raskin P, Klaff L, Bergenstal R, Halle JP, Donley D, Mecca T. A 16-week comparison of the novel insulin analog insulin glargine (HOE 901) and NPH human insulin used with insulin lispro in patients with type 1 diabetes. *Diabetes Care*. 2000;23:1666-1671.

64. Rosenstock J, Park G, Zimmerman J. Basal insulin glargine (HOE 901) versus NPH insulin in patients with type 1 diabetes on multiple daily insulin regimens. *Diabetes Care*. 2000;23:1137-1142.

65. Pieber TR, Eugene-Jolchine I, Derobert E. Efficacy and safety of HOE 901 versus NPH insulin in patients with type 1 diabetes. *Diabetes Care*. 2000;23: 157-162.

66. Witthaus E, Stewart J, Bradley C. Treatment satisfaction and psychological well-being with insulin glargine compared with NPH in patients with type 1 diabetes. *Diabet Med*. 2001;18:619-625.

67. Roach P, Strack T, Arora V, Zhao Z. Improved glycaemic control with the use of self-prepared mixtures of insulin lispro and insulin lispro protamine suspension in patients with types 1 and 2 diabetes. *Int J Clin Pract*. 2001;55:177-182.

68. Tamas G, Marre M, Astorga R, et al. Glycaemic control in type 1 diabetic patients using optimised insulin aspart or human insulin in a randomised multinational study. *Diabetes Res Clin Pract*. 2001;54:105-114.

69. Tsui E, Barnie A, Ross S, Parks R, Zinman B. Intensive insulin therapy with insulin lispro. *Diabetes Care*. 2001;24:1722-1727.

70. Bode BW, Strange P. Efficacy, safety, and pump compatibility of insulin aspart used in continuous subcutaneous insulin infusion therapy in patients with type 1 diabetes. *Diabetes Care*. 2001;24:69-72.

71. Rossetti P, Pampanelli S, Costa E, Torlone E, Brunetti P, Bolli G. A three-month comparison between multiple daily NPH and once daily glargine insulin administration in intensive replacement of basal insulin in type 1 diabetes mellitus. *Diabetes*. 2002;51(suppl 2):A54.

72. Boehm BO, et al. Premixed insulin aspart 30 vs premixed human insulin 30/70 twice daily. *Diabet Med*. 2002;19:393-399.

73. Seigler DE, Olsson GM, Skyler JS. Morning versus bedtime isophane insulin in type 2 (non-insulin dependent) diabetes mellitus. *Diabet Med*. 1992;9:826-833.

74. Groop LC, Widen E, Ekstrand A, et al. Morning or bedtime NPH insulin combined with sulfonylurea in treatment of NIDDM. *Diabetes Care*. 1992;15:831-834.

75. Taylor R, Davies R, Fox C, Sampson M, Weaver JU, Wood L. Appropriate insulin regimes for type 2 diabetes. *Diabetes Care*. 2000;23:1612-1618.

76. Tindall H, Bodansky HJ, Strickland M, Wales JK. A strategy for selection of elderly type 2 diabetic patients for insulin therapy, and a comparison of two insulin preparations. *Diabet Med*. 1988;5:533-536.

77. Paterson KR, Wilson M, Kesson CM, et al. Comparison of basal and prandial insulin therapy in patients with secondary failure of sulfonylurea therapy. *Diabet Med*. 1991;8:40-43.

78. Soneru IL, Agrawal L, Murphy JC, Lawrence AM, Abraira C. Comparison of morning or bedtime insulin with and without glyburide in secondary sulfonylurea failure. *Diabetes Care*. 1993;16:896-901.

79. Taylor R, Foster B, Kyne-Grzebalski D, Vanderpump M. Insulin regimens for the non-insulin dependent. *Diabet Med*. 1994;11:551-557.

80. Saudek CD, Duckwonk WC, Giobbie-Hurder A, et al. Implantable insulin pump vs multiple-dose insulin for non-insulin-dependent diabetes mellitus: a randomized clinical trial. *JAMA*. 1996;276:1322-1327.

81. Bastyr EJ 3rd, Stuart CA, Brodows RG, et al. Therapy focused on lowering postprandial glucose, not fasting glucose, may be superior for lowering HbA1c: IOEZ Study Group. *Diabetes Care*. 2000;23:1236-1241.

82. Bastyr EJ 3rd, Huang Y, Brunelle RL, Vignati L, Cox DJ, Kotsamos JG. Factors associated with nocturnal hypoglycaemia among patients with type 2 diabetes new to insulin therapy. *Diabetes Obes Metab*. 2000; 2:39-46.

83. Fritsche A, Schweitzer MA, Haring H. Improved glycemic control and reduced nocturnal hypoglycemia in patients with type 2 diabetes with morning administration of insulin glargine compared with NPH insulin. *Diabetes*. 2002;51(suppl 2):A54.

84. Lean ME, Ng LL, Tennison BR. Interval between insulin injection and eating in relation to blood glucose control in adult diabetics. *BMJ (Clin Res Ed)*. 1985; 290:105-108.

85. Sackey AH, Jefferson IG. Interval between insulin injection and breakfast in diabetes. *Arch Dis Child*. 1994;71:248-250.

86. Stades AM, Hoekstra JB, van der Tweed I, Erkelens DW, Holleman F, STABILITY Study Group. Additional lunchtime basal insulin during insulin lispro intensive therapy in a randomized, multicenter, crossover study in adults. *Diabetes Care*. 2002;25:712-717.

87. Tunbridge FK, et al. A comparison of human ultralente- and lente-based twice-daily injection regimens. *Diabet Med*. 1989;6:496-501.

88. Bolli GB, Owens DR. Insulin glargine. *Lancet*. 2000; 356:443-445.

89. Porcellati F, Rossetti P, Fanelli CG, Scionti L, Brunetti P, Bolli GB. Glargine vs NPH as basal insulin in intensive treatment of T1DM given lispro at meals. *Diabetes*. 2002;51(suppl 2):A53.

90. Kelly JL, Trence DL, Hirsch IB. Rapid decrease in clinically significant hypoglycemia with insulin glargine. *Diabetes*. 2002;51:A123.

91. Hayward RA, Manning WG, Kaplan SH, Wagner EH, Greenfield S. Starting insulin therapy in patients with type 2 diabetes. *JAMA*. 1997;278:1663-1669.

92. United Kingdom Prospective Diabetes Study 24: a 6-year, randomized, controlled trial comparing sulfonylurea, insulin, and metformin therapy in patients with newly diagnosed type 2 diabetes that could not be controlled with diet therapy. *Ann Intern Med*. 1998;128:165-175.

93. Wright A, Burden AC, Paisey RB, et al. Sulfonylurea inadequacy. *Diabetes Care*. 2002;25:330-336.

94. Turner RC, Cull CA, Frighi V, Holman RR. Glycemic control with diet, sulfonylurea, metformin, or insulin in patients with type 2 diabetes mellitus. *JAMA*. 1999;281:2005-2012.

95. Shichiri M, Kishikawa H, Ohkubo Y, Wake N. Long-term results of the Kumamoto Study on optimal diabetes control in type 2 diabetic patients. *Diabetes Care*. 2000;23(suppl 2):B21-B29.

96. Ohkubo Y, Kishikawa H, Arski E, et al. Intensive insulin therapy prevents the progression of diabetic microvascular complications in Japanese patients with non-insulin-dependent diabetes mellitus. *Diabetes Res Clin Pract*. 1995;28:103-117.

97. Chow CC, Tsang LW, Sorensen JP, Cochram CS. Comparison of insulin with or without continuation of oral hypoglycemic agents in the treatment of secondary failure in NIDDM patients. *Diabetes Care*. 1995; 18:307-314.

98. van der Does FE, de Neeling JN, Snoek FJ, et al. Randomized study of two different target levels of glycemic control within the acceptable range in type 2 diabetes. *Diabetes Care*. 1998;21:2085-2093.

99. Dunbar JM, Madden PM, Gleeson DT, Fiad TM, McKenna TJ. Premixed insulin preparations in pen syringes maintain glycemic control and are preferred by patients. *Diabetes Care*. 1994;17:874-878.

100. Small M, MacRury S, Boal A, Peterson KR, MacCuish AC. Comparison of conventional twice daily subcutaneous insulin administration and a multiple injection regimen (using the NovoPen) in insulin-dependent diabetes mellitus. *Diabetes Res*. 1988;8:85-89.

101. Saurbrey N, Arnold-Larson S, Moller-Jensen B, Kuhl C. Comparison of continuous subcutaneous insulin infusion with multiple insulin injections using the NovoPen. *Diabet Med*. 1988;5:150-153.

102. Murray DP, Keenan P, Gayer E, et al. A randomized trial of the efficacy and acceptability of a pen injector. *Diabet Med.* 1988;5:750-754.
103. Chen HS, Hwu CM, Kwok CF, et al. Clinical response and patient acceptance of a prefilled, disposable insulin pen injector for insulin-treated diabetes. *Zhonghua Yi Xue Za Zhi (Taipei).* 1999;62:455-460.
104. Groop L, Harno K, Tolppanen EM. The combination of insulin and sulfonylurea in the treatment of secondary drug failure in patients with type II diabetes. *Acta Endocrinol (Copenh).* 1984;106:97-101.
105. Groop L, Hano K, Nikkila EA, Pelkonan R, Tolppanen EM. Transient effect of the combination of insulin and sulfonylurea (glibenclamide) on glycemic control in non-insulin dependent diabetics poorly controlled with insulin alone. *Acta Med Scand.* 1985;217:33-39.
106. Samanta A, Burden AC, Kinghorn HA. A comparative study of sulfonylurea and insulin therapy in non insulin dependent diabetics who had failed on diet therapy alone. *Diabetes Res.* 1987;4:183-185.
107. Schade DS, Mitchell WJ, Griego G. Addition of sulfonylurea to insulin treatment in poorly controlled type II diabetes. *JAMA.* 1987;257:2441-2445.
108. Kitabchi AE, Soria AG, Radparvar A, Lawson-Grant V. Combined therapy of insulin and tolazamide decreases insulin requirement and serum triglycerides in obese patients with noninsulin-dependent diabetes mellitus. *Am J Med Sci.* 1987;294:10-14.
109. Holman RR, Steemson J, Turner RC. Sulphonylurea failure in type 2 diabetes. *Diabet Med.* 1987;4:457-462.
110. Stenman S, Groop PH, Saloranta C, Totterman KJ, Fyhrqvist F, Groop L. Effects of the combination of insulin and glibenclamide in type 2 (non-insulin-dependent) diabetic patients with secondary failure to oral hypoglycaemic agents. *Diabetologia.* 1988;31:206-213.
111. Lewitt MS, Yu VK, Rennie GC, et al. Effects of combined insulin-sulfonylurea therapy in type II patients. *Diabetes Care.* 1989;12:379-383.
112. Riddle MC, Hart JS, Bouma DJ, Phillipson BE, Youker G. Efficacy of bedtime NPH insulin with daytime sulfonylurea for subpopulation of type II diabetic subjects. *Diabetes Care.* 1989;12:623-629.
113. Vigneri R, Trischitta V, Italia S, Mazzanno S, Rebuazzo MA, Squatrito S. Treatment of NIDDM patients with secondary failure to glyburide. *Diabet Metab.* 1991;17(1 pt 2):232-234.
114. Trischitta V, Italia S, Mazzarino S, et al. Comparison of combined therapies in treatment of secondary failure to glyburide. *Diabetes Care.* 1992;15:539-542.
115. Ravnik-Oblak M, Mrevlje F. Insulin versus a combination of insulin and sulfonylurea in the treatment of NIDDM patients with secondary oral failure. *Diabetes Res Clin Pract.* 1995;30:27-35.
116. Feinglos MN, Thacker CR, Lobaugh B, et al. Combination insulin and sulfonylurea therapy in insulin-requiring type 2 diabetes mellitus. *Diabetes Res Clin Pract.* 1998;39:193-199.
117. Robinson AC, Burke J, Robinson S, Johnston DG, Elkeles RS. The effects of metformin on glycemic control and serum lipids in insulin-treated NIDDM patients with suboptimal metabolic control. *Diabetes Care.* 1998;21:701-705.
118. Lopez-Alvarenga JC, Aguilar-Salinas CA, Velasco-Perez ML, et al. Acarbose vs bedtime NPH insulin in the treatment of secondary failures to sulfonylurea-metformin therapy in type 2 diabetes mellitus. *Diabetes Obes Metab.* 1999;1:29-35.
119. Fritsche A, Schmulling RM, Haring HU, Stumvoll M. Intensive insulin therapy combined with metformin in obese type 2 diabetic patients. *Acta Diabetol.* 2000;37:13-18.
120. Ponssen HH, Elte JW, Wheat P, Schouten JP, Bets D. Combined metformin and insulin therapy for patients with type 2 diabetes mellitus. *Clin Ther.* 2000;22:709-718.
121. Osei K, O'Dorisio TM, Falko JM. Concomitant insulin and sulfonylurea therapy in patients with type II diabetes. *Am J Med.* 1984;77:1002-1009.
122. Falko JM, Osei K. Combination insulin/glyburide therapy in type II diabetes mellitus. *Am J Med.* 1985;79:92-101.
123. Quatraro A, Consoli G, Cariello A, Giugliano D. Combined insulin and sulfonylurea therapy in non-insulin-dependent diabetics with secondary failure to oral drugs: a one year follow-up. *Diabet Metab.* 1986;12:315-318.
124. Mauerhoff T, Ketelslegers JM, Lambert AE. Effect of glibenclamide in insulin-treated diabetic patients with a residual insulin secretion. *Diabet Metab.* 1986;12:34-38.
125. Gutniak M, Karlander SG, Efendic S. Glyburide decreases insulin requirement, increases beta-cell response to mixed meal, and does not affect insulin sensitivity. *Diabetes Care.* 1987;10:545-554.
126. Reich A, Abraira C, Lawrence AM. Combined glyburide and insulin therapy in type II diabetes. *Diabetes Res.* 1987;6:99-104.
127. Bachmann W, Lotz N, Mehnert H, Rosak C, Schoffling K. [Effectiveness of combined treatment with glibenclamide and insulin in secondary sulfonylurea failure: a controlled multicenter double-blind clinical trial]. *Dtsch Med Wochenschr.* 1988;113:631-636.
128. Casner PR. Insulin-glyburide combination therapy for non-insulin-dependent diabetes mellitus. *Clin Pharmacol Ther.* 1988;44:594-603.
129. Lawrence AM, Abraira C. New modalities in diabetes treatment. *Am J Med.* 1988;85:153-158.
130. Lins PE, Lundblads S, Perrson-Trotzig E, Adamson U. Glibenclamide improves the response to insulin treatment in non-insulin-dependent diabetics with second failure to sulfonylurea therapy. *Acta Med Scand.* 1988;223:171-179.
131. Klein W. Sulfonylurea-metformin-combination versus sulfonylurea-insulin-combination in secondary failures of sulfonylurea monotherapy. *Diabet Metab.* 1991;17(1 pt 2):235-240.
132. Groop L, Widen E. Treatment strategies for secondary sulfonylurea failure. *Diabet Metab.* 1991;17(1 pt 2):218-223.
133. Lebovitz HE. Insulin secretagogues: old and new. *Diabetes Rev.* 1999;7:139-153.
134. Riddle M, Hart J, Bingham P, Garrison C, McDaniel P. Combined therapy for obese type 2 diabetes. *Am J Med Sci.* 1992;303:151-156.
135. Chiasson JL, Josse RG, Hunt JA, et al. The efficacy of acarbose in the treatment of patients with non-insulin-dependent diabetes mellitus. *Ann Intern Med.* 1994;121:928-935.
136. Shank ML, Del Prato S, DeFronzo RA. Bedtime insulin/daytime glipizide. *Diabetes.* 1995;44:165-172.
137. Clauson P, Karlander S, Steen L, Effendic S. Daytime glibenclamide and bedtime NPH insulin compared to intensive insulin treatment in secondary sulfonylurea failure. *Diabet Med.* 1996;13:471-477.
138. Wolffenbuttel BH, Sels JP, Rondas-Colbeas GJ, Menheere PP, Nieuwanhuijzen Krusaman AC. Comparison of different insulin regimens in elderly patients with NIDDM. *Diabetes Care.* 1996;19:1326-1332.
139. Colwell JA. The feasibility of intensive insulin management in non-insulin-dependent diabetes mellitus. *Ann Intern Med.* 1996;124(1 pt 2):131-135.
140. Relimpio F, Pumer A, Losada F, Mangas MA, Acosta D, Astorga R. Adding metformin versus insulin dose increase in insulin-treated but poorly controlled type 2 diabetes mellitus. *Diabet Med.* 1998;15:997-1002.
141. Niazi R, Muzaffar Z. Comparison of bedtime NPH insulin or metformin combined with glibenclamide in secondary sulfonylurea failure in obese type II (NIDDM) patients. *J Pak Med Assoc.* 1998;48:336-338.
142. Kelley DE, Bidot P, Freidman Z, et al. Efficacy and safety of acarbose in insulin-treated patients with type 2 diabetes. *Diabetes Care.* 1998;21:2056-2061.
143. Riddle MC, Schneider J. Beginning insulin treatment of obese patients with evening 70/30 insulin plus glimepiride versus insulin alone. *Diabetes Care.* 1998;21:1052-1057.
144. Yki-Jarvinen H, Ruysy L, Nikkila K, Tulokas T, Vanamo R, Heikkilla M. Comparison of bedtime insulin regimens in patients with type 2 diabetes mellitus. *Ann Intern Med.* 1999;130:389-396.
145. Aviles-Santa L, Sinding J, Raskin P. Effects of metformin in patients with poorly controlled, insulin-treated type 2 diabetes mellitus. *Ann Intern Med.* 1999;131:182-188.
146. Bastyr EJ 3rd, Johnston ME, Trautmann ME, Anderson JH Jr, Vignati L. Insulin lispro in the treatment of patients with type 2 diabetes mellitus after oral agent failure. *Clin Ther.* 1999;21:1703-1714.
147. Wulffele MG, Kooy A, Lehert P, et al. Discontinuation of metformin in type 2 diabetes patients treated with insulin. *Neth J Med.* 2002;60:249-252.
148. Yki-Jarvinen H. Combination therapies with insulin in type 2 diabetes. *Diabetes Care.* 2001;24:758-767.
149. Frazier LM, Malrow CD, Alexander LT Jr, et al. Need for insulin therapy in type II diabetes mellitus. *Arch Intern Med.* 1987;147:1085-1089.
150. Inzucchi SE. Oral antihyperglycemic therapy for type 2 diabetes: scientific review. *JAMA.* 2002;287:360-372.
151. Strowig SM, Aviles-Santa ML, Raskin P. Comparison of insulin monotherapy and combination therapy with insulin and metformin or insulin and troglitazone in type 2 diabetes. *Diabetes Care.* 2002;25:1691-1698.
152. Delea T, Hagiwara M, Edelsberg J, et al. Exposure to glitazone antidiabetics and risk of heart failure among persons with type 2 diabetes. *J Am Coll Cardiol.* 2002;39(suppl A):184A.
153. Abraira C, Colwell JA, Nuttall FQ, et al. Veterans Affairs Cooperative Study on glycemic control and complications in type II diabetes (VA CSDM). *Diabetes Care.* 1995;18:1113-1123.
154. Henry RR, Gumbiner B, Ditzler T, Wallace P, Lyon R, Glauber NS. Intensive conventional insulin therapy for type II diabetes. *Diabetes Care.* 1993;16:21-31.
155. Pickup J, Mattock M, Kerry S. Glycaemic control with continuous subcutaneous insulin infusion compared with intensive insulin injections in patients with type 1 diabetes. *BMJ.* 2002;324:705.
156. Gabbe SG, Holing E, Temple P, Brown ZA. Benefits, risks, costs, and patient satisfaction associated with insulin pump therapy for the pregnancy complicated by type 1 diabetes mellitus. *Am J Obstet Gynecol.* 2000;182:1283-1291.
157. Thompson DM, Kozak SE, Sheps S. Insulin adjustment by a diabetes nurse educator improves glucose control in insulin-requiring diabetic patients. *CMAJ.* 1999;161:959-962.
158. Biermann E, Dietrich W, Standl E. Telecare of diabetic patients with intensified insulin therapy. *Stud Health Technol Inform.* 2000;77:327-332.
159. Peters A, Rubsamen M, Jacob U, Look D, Scriba PC. Clinical evaluation of decision support system for insulin-dose adjustment in IDDM. *Diabetes Care.* 1991;14:875-880.
160. Schrezenmeir J, Dirting K, Papazov P. Controlled multicenter study on the effect of computer assistance in intensive insulin therapy of type 1 diabetics. *Comput Methods Programs Biomed.* 2002;69:97-114.
161. Holmboe ES. Oral antihyperglycemic therapy for type 2 diabetes: clinical applications. *JAMA.* 2002;287:373-376.
162. Johnson JA, Majumdar SR, Simpson SH, Toth EL. Decreased mortality associated with the use of metformin compared with sulfonylurea monotherapy in type 2 diabetes. *Diabetes Care.* 2002;25:2244-2248.
163. *Practical Insulin: A Handbook for Prescribing Providers.* Alexandria, Va: American Diabetes Association; 2002.

NOTES

NOTES

NOTES

NOTES

NOTES

NOTES

Please address inquiries on bulk subscriptions and permission to reproduce selections from this White Paper to Medletter Associates, Inc., 632 Broadway, 11th Floor, New York, NY 10012. The editors are interested in receiving your comments at Editors@HopkinsWhitePapers.com or the above address but regret that they cannot answer letters of any sort personally.

ISBN 0-929661-92-3
ISSN 1542-1449
Tenth Printing
Printed in the United States of America

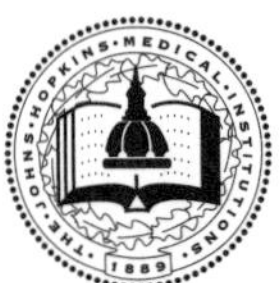

The Johns Hopkins White Papers are published yearly by Medletter Associates, Inc.

Visit our Web site for information on Johns Hopkins Health After 50 publications, which include White Papers on specific disorders, home medical encyclopedias, consumer reference guides to drugs and medical tests, and our monthly newsletter *The Johns Hopkins Medical Letter: Health After 50.*
www.HopkinsAfter50.com

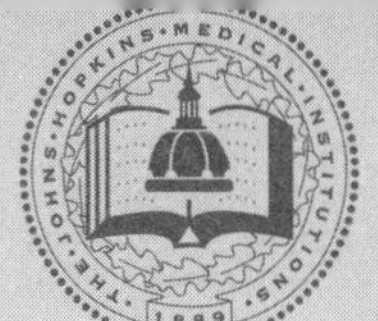

The 2004 White Papers

64B60M

Take Control of Your Medical Condition

Visit us online at www.HopkinsAfter50.com

YES, I've placed a check mark next to the White Paper(s) I'd like to receive for $24.95 each. Annual updates on each subject that I have chosen will be offered to me by announcement card. I need do nothing if I want the update to be sent to me automatically. If I do not want it, I will return the announcement card marked "cancel." I may cancel at any time. (Please add $2.95 for domestic, $4.95 for Canadian, and $15.00 for foreign orders to your total to cover shipping and handling.) (Florida residents add sales tax.)

✔ **Please put a check mark next to the White Paper(s) you wish to order.**

- 001040 ❑ Arthritis $24.95
- 003046 ❑ Coronary Heart Disease $24.95
- 004044 ❑ Depression and Anxiety $24.95
- 005041 ❑ Diabetes $24.95
- 006049 ❑ Hypertension and Stroke $24.95
- 007047 ❑ Nutrition and Weight Control for Longevity $24.95
- 008045 ❑ Prostate Disorders $24.95
- 010041 ❑ Digestive Disorders $24.95
- 011049 ❑ Vision $24.95
- 012047 ❑ Back Pain & Osteoporosis $24.95
- 015040 ❑ Memory $24.95
- 019042 ❑ Lung Disorders $24.95
- 020040 ❑ Heart Attack Prevention $24.95

METHOD OF PAYMENT: (U.S. funds only) ❑ VISA ❑ Check Enclosed ❑ MasterCard ❑ Bill Me

Name

Address

City State Zip

Credit Card # Exp. Date

Signature Date

Money Back Guarantee: If for any reason, you are not satisfied after receipt of your publications, return your purchase within 30 days for a full refund.

Detach and mail this card back to The Johns Hopkins White Papers, P.O. Box 420083, Palm Coast, FL 32142

The 2004 White Papers

64B60M

Take Control of Your Medical Condition

Visit us online at www.HopkinsAfter50.com

YES, I've placed a check mark next to the White Paper(s) I'd like to receive for $24.95 each. Annual updates on each subject that I have chosen will be offered to me by announcement card. I need do nothing if I want the update to be sent to me automatically. If I do not want it, I will return the announcement card marked "cancel." I may cancel at any time. (Please add $2.95 for domestic, $4.95 for Canadian, and $15.00 for foreign orders to your total to cover shipping and handling.) (Florida residents add sales tax.)

✔ **Please put a check mark next to the White Paper(s) you wish to order.**

- 001040 ❑ Arthritis $24.95
- 003046 ❑ Coronary Heart Disease $24.95
- 004044 ❑ Depression and Anxiety $24.95
- 005041 ❑ Diabetes $24.95
- 006049 ❑ Hypertension and Stroke $24.95
- 007047 ❑ Nutrition and Weight Control for Longevity $24.95
- 008045 ❑ Prostate Disorders $24.95
- 010041 ❑ Digestive Disorders $24.95
- 011049 ❑ Vision $24.95
- 012047 ❑ Back Pain & Osteoporosis $24.95
- 015040 ❑ Memory $24.95
- 019042 ❑ Lung Disorders $24.95
- 020040 ❑ Heart Attack Prevention $24.95

METHOD OF PAYMENT: (U.S. funds only) ❑ VISA ❑ Check Enclosed ❑ MasterCard ❑ Bill Me

Name

Address

City State Zip

Credit Card # Exp. Date

Signature Date

Money Back Guarantee: If for any reason, you are not satisfied after receipt of your publications, return your purchase within 30 days for a full refund.

Detach and mail this card back to The Johns Hopkins White Papers, P.O. Box 420083, Palm Coast, FL 32142

Johns Hopkins White Papers

Fold along this line and tape closed

NO POSTAGE NECESSARY IF MAILED IN THE UNITED STATES

BUSINESS REPLY MAIL
FIRST-CLASS MAIL PERMIT NO. 86 FLAGLER BEACH FL

POSTAGE WILL BE PAID BY ADDRESSEE

THE JOHNS HOPKINS WHITE PAPERS
PO BOX 420083
PALM COAST FL 32142-9264

Johns Hopkins White Papers

Fold along this line and tape closed

NO POSTAGE NECESSARY IF MAILED IN THE UNITED STATES

BUSINESS REPLY MAIL
FIRST-CLASS MAIL PERMIT NO. 86 FLAGLER BEACH FL

POSTAGE WILL BE PAID BY ADDRESSEE

THE JOHNS HOPKINS WHITE PAPERS
PO BOX 420083
PALM COAST FL 32142-9264

2004 WHITE PAPER TITLES

ARTHRITIS 2004 - Covers three common forms of arthritis - osteoarthritis, rheumatoid arthritis, and gout - as well as two other rheumatic diseases: fibromyalgia syndrome and bursitis.

CORONARY HEART DISEASE 2004 - Discusses four problems resulting from coronary heart disease: heart attacks, angina, cardiac arrhythmias, and heart failure.

DEPRESSION and ANXIETY 2004 - Includes major depression, dysthymia, atypical depression, bipolar disorder, seasonal affective disorder, panic disorder, generalized anxiety disorder, obsessive-compulsive disorder, post-traumatic stress disorder, and phobic disorders.

DIABETES 2004 - Shows you how to manage your diabetes and avoid complications such as foot problems and vision changes. Reviews the latest tools for monitoring your blood glucose and the newest medications for controlling it.

DIGESTIVE DISORDERS 2004 - Covers gastroesophageal reflux disease, peptic ulcers, dysphagia, achalasia, Barrett's esophagus, esophageal spasm and stricture, gastritis, gallstones, diarrhea, constipation, Crohn's disease, ulcerative colitis, and colon cancer.

HYPERTENSION and STROKE 2004 - Explains how to treat your high blood pressure and prevent it from harming your health. Also covers the two forms of stroke: ischemic stroke and hemorrhagic stroke.

BACK PAIN and OSTEOPOROSIS 2004 - Addresses back pain due to sprains, strains, and spasms; degenerative changes of the spinal bones and disks; disk herniation; and spinal stenosis. Also covers osteoporosis, a common cause of fractures in the spine and hip.

LUNG DISORDERS 2004 - Includes information on emphysema and chronic bronchitis (together referred to as chronic obstructive pulmonary disease or COPD), asthma, pneumonia, tuberculosis, lung cancer, and sleep apnea.

MEMORY 2004 - Tells you how to keep your memory sharp as you get older, and how to recognize the symptoms of age-associated memory impairment, mild cognitive impairment, and illnesses such as Alzheimer's disease and vascular dementia.

NUTRITION and WEIGHT CONTROL for LONGEVITY 2004 - Gives you the information you need to eat a healthy diet and keep your weight under control. Also explains what to do when the pounds just don't seem to budge.

PROSTATE DISORDERS 2004 - Helps you decide among the various treatment options for prostate cancer, benign prostatic hyperplasia, and prostatitis.

VISION 2004 - Reviews the current knowledge on cataracts, glaucoma, age-related macular degeneration, and diabetic retinopathy. Also discusses ways to cope with low vision.

HEART ATTACK PREVENTION 2004 - Provides up-to-date strategies for preventing a first heart attack, including identifying possible risk factors, the latest screening tests, risk-reducing lifestyle measures, and medications for controlling cholesterol.